Mind Matters
in Children

Mind Matters
in Children

Kenneth Lyen

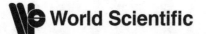
World Scientific

NEW JERSEY · LONDON · SINGAPORE · BEIJING · SHANGHAI · HONG KONG · TAIPEI · CHENNAI · TOKYO

Published by

World Scientific Publishing Co. Pte. Ltd.

5 Toh Tuck Link, Singapore 596224

USA office: 27 Warren Street, Suite 401-402, Hackensack, NJ 07601

UK office: 57 Shelton Street, Covent Garden, London WC2H 9HE

Library of Congress Cataloging-in-Publication Data
Names: Lyen, Kenneth, author.
Title: Mind matters in children : nil / Kenneth Lyen.
Description: 1st edition. | Hackensack, NJ : World Scientific, [2023] |
    Includes bibliographical references and index.
Identifiers: LCCN 2022041395 | ISBN 9789811252402 (hardcover) |
    ISBN 9789811253324 (paperback) | ISBN 9789811252419 (ebook for institutions) |
    ISBN 9789811252426 (ebook for individuals)
Subjects: LCSH: Child psychology. | Child development. | Mind and body.
Classification: LCC BF721 .L94 2023 | DDC 155.4--dc23/eng/20221017
LC record available at https://lccn.loc.gov/2022041395

British Library Cataloguing-in-Publication Data
A catalogue record for this book is available from the British Library.

For any available supplementary material, please visit
https://www.worldscientific.com/worldscibooks/10.1142/12727#t=suppl

Typeset by Stallion Press
Email: enquiries@stallionpress.com

Printed in Singapore

About Kenneth Lyen

Dr Kenneth Lyen graduated from Oxford University Medical School before undertaking specialist paediatric training at the Great Ormond Street Hospital for Children in London, and the Children's Hospital of Philadelphia. Upon his return to Singapore, he was appointed senior lecturer and consultant at the National University of Singapore.

He founded three special schools for disabled and autistic children, namely the Rainbow Centre at Margaret Drive (1987), the Rainbow Centre at Yishun Park (1995), and the Rainbow Centre at Woodlands (2018). For his work with disabled children, he received the Public Service Medal in 1997 and the Public Service Star in 2022. He remains on the board of management for the Rainbow Centre.

Dr Lyen has co-authored many books on paediatrics, parenting, creativity, and education. He has published original research papers on paediatric endocrinology, neurology, and infectious diseases, and medical review articles. He has previously served on the editorial board of the *Singapore Medical Journal*, *Motherhood*, and *Young Families*.

Dedication

This book is dedicated to:

My wife, Dr Huang Yuen Chin
My son Dr Stephen Lyen, his wife Dr Claudia Hon, and their children Max and Chloe
My daughter Claire Lyen, her husband Benjamin Phipps, and their children Elizabeth, Joseph and Jude
My sons Paul and Brian

They have all been a tremendous inspiration for me to write this book.

Foreword

This book by Dr Kenneth Lyen is indeed timely. The world is increasingly complex for our children to navigate, and with the many stresses on them, children suffering from anxiety and depression is a condition that parents, teachers and health providers must be sensitive to and be able to recognise. The mental health of children and youth was brought even more to the fore by the Covid pandemic, with an increased spike of teenage suicides. For children with neuro-developmental issues, the impact of the pressures on them are even more so.

As a parent to special children with learning differences and other developmental issues, I have first hand experience of how critically important it is for our children's development and happiness that their conditions are recognised early so they can receive appropriate interventions, including the school's support. These children often appear normal, but because of learning and socialisation issues, they don't perform well in school, causing them to be labelled as poor students. Sometimes parents, without guidance, also do not recognise their children's struggles, and perhaps further pressure them instead of seeking help and giving them the support that they need. Worse is that the children believe that about themselves and lose confidence, impacting them deeply in every aspect of their lives well into the future.

As a paediatrician, I have also witnessed the anxiety and depression in children who struggled in school and at home, and felt utterly alone, distraught and angry, because no one — parents included — can see their pain. For some children, this further presents as behaviour issues in school and they are labelled as trouble makers, while the root cause is something that can be addressed. As health providers and teachers for children, we must have a high index of suspicion and be highly sensitive to signs and symptoms of anxiety, depression and clues of neuro-developmental conditions. We need to probe and make enquiry into school performance and any behaviour issues in school early on as part of our regular developmental assessment. Regrettably, we are often not sufficiently trained in this area.

Dr Lyen's book gives us the additional knowledge and insight that enable us to help children get early diagnosis and intervention and set the trajectory of their lives in a positive direction, as they deserve. I am grateful for this additional resource and would highly recommend it for all health providers and teachers. And of course, for parents.

Dr Mary Ann Tsao

Preface

This book is about the mental health of children.

Our mind is one of the most extraordinary wonders of mankind! We use it to think critically and creatively. It stores our treasured memories, helps us to make friends and look after our loved ones, and it can transform our impossible dreams into reality.

Sometimes we encounter glitches in our life's journey. The brain may not advance as fast as expected. We may have difficulty socialising, unable to concentrate on our work, have problems speaking, reading and writing, lose our memory, and we may become depressed and even suicidal.

This book delves into both the normal as well as the abnormal functioning of the human mind. It also examines recent developments in neuroscience and how it is helping to reshape our concepts of thinking, creativity and consciousness.

The book is timely because of the recent surge in interest of how the human mind works during the COVID-19 pandemic where there has been a dramatic worldwide increase in mental problems brought about by isolation, economic slowdown, unemployment, and loss of our loved ones. It also looks at how digital technology has affected children and caused gaming addiction.

I was inspired to pen this book because of my own experiences. I have gained a wealth of knowledge through starting three schools for disabled and autistic children under the Rainbow Centre, running a paediatric clinic and caring for countless children with normal and delayed development. I have also taught medical students throughout the years, as well as helped to co-author many books and articles on child development and education. All these experiences are collected into this book.

I will look at normal and exceptional brain functioning from a medical and neuroscience perspective. By doing so, I hope to remove some of the stigma associated with psychological conditions, while simultaneously revealing greater insights into the astounding workings of the human mind.

This book is aimed at parents, teachers, doctors, nurses, psychologists, social workers, therapists, medical and psychology students, and everyone who is fascinated by the human mind.

Yes indeed, the mind matters!

Kenneth Lyen
September 2022

Acknowledgements

I am extremely grateful for the following for reading my manuscript and making important suggestions, correcting my mistakes, editing and clarifying the text:

Dr Paras Sharma, Consultant Neurodevelopmental and Mental Health Paediatrician
Epsom and St Helier University Hospitals, UK.

Dr Denise Au Eong
Tan Tock Seng Hospital, Singapore.

Dr Christopher Chew, Consultant Cardiologist
Mt Elizabeth Medical Centre, Singapore.

Dr Lee Woon Kwang, Consultant Paediatrician
Gleneagles Hospital, Singapore.

Dr Sonny Chong, Consultant Paediatric Gastroenterologist
Epsom and St Helier University Hospitals, UK.

Dr Mary Ann Tsao, Pediatrician
I would like to thank Dr Mary Ann Tsao for writing the foreword. She is a mother of two children with learning difficulties, and was a major supporter helping to establish the Rainbow Centre for developmentally delayed and autistic children.

Important Note

Please check with your healthcare contact, psychologist, therapist, educationalist, or medical practitioner to ensure that the advice given in this book are appropriate for your child.

Contents

1 Child development: The first year

Introduction

"I'm worried that my one-year-old is not walking or talking compared to another child of the same age friend who is already so active. What should I do?" asks a parent. Not everyone develops at the same pace, and indeed, there is a wide range in the speed of development among different children, and even the rate within one child can proceed at different tempos. The descriptions below are what an average child is expected to achieve at the given ages.

Definition

Child development is the continuous process of changes in physical, language, intellectual, behavioural, emotional and social functioning from birth to adolescence.

Assessment of child development

In assessing the development of a child, we look for four main categories of development: gross motor, fine motor, speech, and personal-social.

- Gross motor: refers mainly to the muscles of the neck, the back and the lower limbs involved in rolling over, sitting, crawling, standing, walking and jumping.
- Fine motor: This refers to the muscles of the hands, fingers and wrists; these are involved in activities such as grasping small objects, stacking toy blocks, dressing, drawing and writing.

- Speech: While assessing speech, it is important to first exclude hearing difficulties. Speech assessment involves two major areas: firstly, the receptive ability of the child to interpret the signals encouraging a response, that is, the ability to understand what the tester is trying to promote; secondly, the motor ability of the child to produce the vowel and consonant sounds that make up words.
- Personal-social: This assessment involves seeing how the child responds to parents and strangers. Responses include waving, clapping, and indicating needs or activities such as playing ball, using a cup or spoon, and dressing themselves.

Although the majority of children will achieve the milestones listed below, there is nonetheless quite a wide range in the pace of development. Some will achieve their behaviour-or physical skills at an earlier age while others at a later date. It is safe to say that if a child cannot achieve two or more milestones by the next milestone date, then we can say they might be developmentally delayed. For example if a child of nine months cannot sit unsupported, or a 15-month-old child cannot say "baba" or "mama", we can recommend consultation by a practitioner.

At birth

The first thing that a baby does at birth is cry and take the first breath. The doctor or nurse then proceeds to carry out a full physical examination to make sure that the child is healthy.

The newborn is quite weak, and when held under the chest and belly with the head facing down (ventral suspension), the spine may be slightly curved. The head may droop a little bit, and the arms and legs are flexed slightly. As the baby assumes a sitting position with the arms pulled forwards, the head will loll backwards. When the newborn is more awake, they may respond to their parents' faces and hear them speak.

Primitive reflexes are involuntary motor responses originating in the central nervous system. They usually disappear by three to six months. When held in a half-sitting position at a 45° angle, and the baby's head is suddenly allowed to carefully and safely fall backwards, the infant may be surprised while extending the arms outwards and then bringing them back to the chest. This startle reflex is known as the "Moro reflex". Another primitive reflex is the "sucking reflex", an instinctive sucking action which occurs when you put the mother's nipple, a nursing bottle, or a pacifier into the baby's mouth. When you stroke the corner of the mouth, the baby's head may turn in the direction of the stimulus; this is known as the "rooting reflex". The evolutionary explanation of this reflex is that when the mother's nipple touches the lips, the infant will turn to put it in the mouth, and thereby get some milk.

1-month-old

Developmentally, the 1-month-old is quite similar to the newborn. The baby can turn to light, and if you move your head in front of them, they can follow your face, perhaps a bit more easily than at birth. Indeed, when the mother is breast or bottle feeding, the baby can look at and respond to her face. They might stop whimpering when a parent calls them. Also present at birth is a reflex known as the "grasp reflex", where the 1-month-old baby can grasp your finger using their entire palm when you place your finger into the baby's hand . When pulled to sit, there is still quite a bit of head lolling. All the other primitive reflexes are still present.

2-month-old

The 2-month-old can lift the head when lying prone on the abdomen. They are happy when they see their mother, and their smile appears to be more genuine, and is referred to as a "social smile". The eye tracking is better, and the baby can follow faces and objects more consistently. If you call out to the 2-month-old, they can turn in the direction of your voice. The baby is alert for longer periods of time.

4-month-old

The 4-month-old can roll from front to back, and one should be careful, because rolling over carries a risk of falling onto the floor from a bed or couch. They can bring their hands to the midline, and grasp objects more firmly than a few months earlier. They can use sounds to communicate and their social smile is most engaging.

6-month-old

At 6 months, the baby is becoming quite strong, and can struggle energetically when held in your arms. When pulled to sit, they flex their neck forwards in anticipation of the act. They sit with either minimal or no support, and their spine is quite straight. When lying prone, the arms are extended and their chest can be pushed off the couch. They can lift their leg, grab their foot, and when held standing, the legs can bear their weight without buckling.

The baby's hands are now also more dexterous. They can grasp a large ball with both hands, or a smaller object using a palmar grasp, and they can transfer the object from one hand to the other. A ball rolling more than 5 feet away can be followed by the 6-month-old. A soft sound or voice coming from behind can be heard, and the infant can turn all the way round to locate it. They can babble quite extensively.

9-month-old

The 9-month-old is starting to crawl, pull themselves up to stand, and can cruise around holding furniture. They can begin to pick up small objects with their finger and thumb, which is described as an immature "pincer grasp". Whatever they pick up goes straight into their mouth. They can turn the pages of a board book. Although they can say "mama" or "baba", it can refer indiscriminately to any person around them. Some children can say "bye bye" and wave at you at the same time. When an object is hidden from sight, they know that it continues to exist, and can remove the cover hiding it. This is referred to as "object permanence". At this age, the child may be upset when a caregiver leaves them alone, a situation described as "separation anxiety". When holding a baby upright, and then you quickly but gently rotate the body forward and downward, to simulate falling, the infant will automatically extend their arms forwards trying to break the fall. This is known as the "parachute reflex".

12-month-old

The first birthday is an important celebration and is an occasion to examine the child closely for developmental milestones. They can pull themselves up to stand more easily, and can walk with one hand held. They can point, shake a rattle, and their pincer grasp is more advanced. "Mama" and "baba" are spoken more accurately, and refers correctly to either mother or father. There may be other single words like "ball" or "dog". Occasionally they can imitate clapping hands or respond to "high five" with a raised hand. They may follow simple commands like "give!" or "come here!" They are now more aware of strangers, and some are frightened by new faces, a phenomenon known as "stranger anxiety".

Red flags

The following are guidelines for showing concern if the child is not doing the following activities at these ages:

2-month-old

- not bringing a hand to the mouth
- not responding to loud sounds
- not focusing on things with the eyes
- never smiling when looking at familiar faces
- never turning head from one side to the other
- limbs are either too stiff or too floppy

4-month-old

- not trying to swipe at, or reach out and grasp toys
- not bringing objects to mouth
- not able to keep head steady when held upright
- not turning round to locate sound or getting startled in response to loud sounds
- not pushing down with legs when placed on a firm surface
- not able to lift head or push up with arms when lying on the abdomen

- not moving eyes in all directions
- not smiling regularly during play

6-month-old

- not able to roll over from stomach to back
- not able to sit (with help)
- not laughing or squealing
- not reacting specially to those taking care of them
- not following objects well with both eyes
- not reaching out for toys
- not bearing weight on the legs
- stiffness or floppiness in limbs that might have been overlooked earlier
- persistence of primitive reflexes (Moro, grasp, rooting)

9-month-old

- not able to stand when supported
- not making any efforts to move around
- not able to sit even with help
- not able to babble or attempt to say single words ("baba", "mama")
- not able to use gestures (e.g. wave hand or shake head)
- not showing preference for people who look after them
- startles easily

12-month-old

- not interested in playing
- not turning to person talking to them, not reacting to loud sounds
- not babbling or making a range of sounds
- not pointing to show what they are interested in
- not crawling or bottom-shuffling (scooting): 25% of normal children do not crawl
- not trying to stand up even when encouraged
- not walking when hand held

When red flags are raised, it is recommended that you consult a doctor to see if there are any medical concerns.

Conclusions

We are often surprised when we follow a child's development. New-borns spend much of their life sleeping, feeding and crying. They then transform at an amazingly fast pace into a smiling, interactive, energetic infant.

We hope that the baby is normal, but we often compare them with relatives' and friends' children of a similar age, and we become worried when the infant may seem slower by comparison. One needs to bear in mind that children develop at different rates. Look at the red flag check list to get some ideas as to whether or not to seek medical help.

Here is some other advice. It is important to interact with your baby, to talk to them, play with them, and calm them down gently when they are upset and crying. All babies will cry, and you will be affected by this. If possible, try to find someone to help you look after the baby while you get some rest. Always remember that safety is a priority, so look out for potential dangers like falling from a bed or couch, cuts with sharp objects, unsafe electrical cables or sockets, leaving a child unattended in a bath tub, etc. Limit the amount of screen time watching television or animated videos on electronic devices to no more than a few minutes per day. Many paediatricians actually recommend zero screen time for the first year or two, and replacing television or mobile phone videos with direct human interaction. Looking after children has been a challenge since time immemorial. Get help if you have difficulty coping.

References

1. Shaw G. Baby's first year. WebMD 2011. https://www.webmd.com/parenting/baby/features/stages-of-development
2. Christiano D. Get ready for all these precious first-year milestones. Healthline 2019. https://www.healthline.com/health/baby/baby-development-stages

3. What To Expect First Year. Baby's development month by month. https://www.whattoexpect.com/first-year/month-by-month/

4. Morin A. Developmental milestones from birth to age 1. Understood https://www.understood.org/articles/en/developmental-milestones-from-birth-to-age-1

5. Mersch J. Infant milestones month to month. eMedicineHealth. https://www.emedicinehealth.com/infant_milestones/article_em.htm

2 Toddler development: 18 months to 5 years

Introduction

Toddlers are children between the ages of 18 months and 5 years. They are growing and developing remarkably quickly, and they are becoming more independent. Sometimes, they want to assert their authority by doing what they want and disobeying their caregivers. This can be a very challenging phase of their lives. Understanding their evolution at each stage can be crucial in guiding them to achieve their fullest potential.

Definition

Toddler development is the continuous process of changes in physical, language, intellectual, behavioural, emotional and social functioning from 18 months to 5 years.

Development does not follow a strict linear timeline, and some areas can progress at different rates. For example, some children's physical development might occur later, while speech and language might advance earlier in others.

18-month-old

The 18-month-old child has been walking for a few months, but they lack coordination and may fall easily. They have started to climb stairs but may need a helping hand. Going down stairs can be a bit difficult at this age.

They may be able to stack a tower of three to four blocks, use a spoon to feed themselves, and drink from a cup. They can use crayons to scribble on paper, and turn the pages of a book, often a few pages at a time. They can look at a story book while listening to it being read, and point to pictures in the book. When asked, their finger might touch that part of the body or a toy animal being referred to. Some can indicate what food or drink they want by pointing at the item.

Often, there is a broad social smile and the 18-month-old can interact affectionately with their caregivers. The vocabulary is rapidly expanding, and they can say 10 or more words, including the command "No!" while shaking their head. They might know the function of certain objects like the use of a spoon, a comb or a toothbrush. They can imitate what adults are doing, such as pretending to wipe the table, and they can engage in pretend play, like feeding a doll. Some are starting to be able to dress themselves, like taking off their shoes but not putting them on, and pulling down but not pulling up their pants.

They love to explore their surrounding environment, but they might prefer to have an adult around. Stranger anxiety may be more evident at this age, and they can become upset more easily, displaying noisy temper tantrums. When going to a new environment, they can become more clingy towards their caregiver.

2-year-old

The 2-year-old can run very well, climb up and down stairs, one step at a time, and they can also climb onto furniture. They can throw, kick and catch a ball. Manual dexterity is getting better, and they can build a tower of six cubes, and turn book pages one at a time. They can remove shoes, socks, and underpants, but have difficulty putting clothes on. When asked to point to body parts like the nose or ears, they can do so more confidently. Their vocabulary has increased to over 50 words, and they can often point to indicate their needs. Some can join two words together like "No more" or "Don't want!" Others can even use their own name to refer to themselves. They can understand simple commands like "Give!", or "Fetch your shoes!" Defiant words like "No!" become more common, and they start to show wilful behaviour, leading to temper tantrums if they do not get what they want.

The toddler can feed themselves with a spoon, but it can be quite messy. They can engage in make-believe play, such as pretending to cook. Socialising becomes more common, but sharing of toys is inconsistent. Their sense of curiosity is enhanced, and they are beginning to explore their environment.

3-year-old

The 3-year-old is very energetic and likes to run and jump. Some can walk up the stairs by themselves and stand on tiptoe. When given a tricycle, they may be able to pedal it. Generally, they can undress themselves by pulling off their shoes and pants, and they can assist in the removal of their vests. A few are able to dress themselves, and some can even do the buttons.

They can be very expressive in their speech, with a vocabulary of about 200 words, and their sentences are at least three words long. By the age of three, they can distinguish between "I", "me", "we", "you", and "mine". Some like talking to themselves, others are really quite noisy and ask a lot of questions beginning with "what", "where", and "who". They can carry on a conversation using sentences. A few have a short fuse, and they shout at or hound their caregivers until they get what they want. When taught, they can sing nursery rhymes, recite and point to some letters of the alphabet. They can name the numbers 1 to 10, but may not appreciate the quantity they represent beyond 1-2-3.

The toddler can sort objects according to their shape or colour, and build a tower of nine blocks, and imitate building a simple bridge with just three blocks. Some children may try to take a toy apart to see how it works. They can copy a circle and a cross, and draw the head of a person with a couple of other facial parts. When given a crayon or paintbrush, some really enjoy their "art". Given a pair of child-safe scissors, they are able to cut paper with it. At this age, their imagination starts to flower.

4-year-old

The vocabulary of a 4-year-old can reach 1,000 words or more, and their sentences can be over four words long. They can listen to and retell stories, and they may recognise letters in their name and even try to write their own name. Some appear to be able to read but more often they have just memorised the word prompted by visual cues on the page. They will know a few numbers, and some might even be able to add $1 + 1 = 2$.

The 4-year-old can walk up and down stairs, climb ladders, run around on tiptoe, and hop on one leg. They can catch a bouncing ball, and ride a tricycle. However, when asked to sit still, they may not be able to do so for more than a couple of minutes. Their fine motor skill is quite well developed, and they can thread beads to make a necklace, and hold a pencil quite firmly for drawing and writing.

They are quite sociable and interact with their peers. Some are quite fast in learning about turn-taking and sharing. The toddler loves doing new things, and engages in dramatic make-believe play. They may display a sense of humour like deliberately misnaming an object or changing the plot when retelling a story. Singing nursery rhymes or reciting a poem from memory can often be heard. If their playmate or sibling is in distress, they will show concern. On occasion, they can argue with others by using words rather than force. Their understanding continues to deepen, and they may know the difference between past, present, and future time.

5-year-old

The 5-year-old is extraordinarily lively. They can run, climb, swing, hop, skip, jump, and even dance to music. They can throw and catch balls and pick up very small objects. They may be able to fully dress and undress themselves. Some are good at tidying up their room at home, but others may need prompting.

They are able to count 1 to 10, add $2 + 2 = 4$, but may have difficulty with subtraction. They can copy a square and a triangle. They can also draw a person with four or more parts (head, trunk, legs, arms), sketch a simple house, and write several letters (A, B, C) and their own name. When colouring a picture, they can stay within the outline. At 5 years old, they may show a preference in using their right or left hand.

They usually love listening to stories being told and try to read story books for children. When asked, they can often retell or act out the stories they have heard. They enjoy hearing songs, jokes and riddles. Socialising with their peers plays an important part of their lives, and they like to make friends and participate in rowdy activities. They can understand many more words, including "because". Some will feel a bit more mature and develop a sense of responsibility in looking after their friends and siblings.

Red flags

At the different ages listed below, failure for the toddler to perform certain expected activities, are red flags that parents, caregivers, and teachers should detect and take action.

18-month-old

- Not able to walk
- Not pointing to show things to others
- Not knowing what familiar things (comb, spoon, crayons) are for
- Not imitating other people's gestures (clap, wave)
- Not able to say at least six words
- Not learning new words
- Not noticing or not being anxious when a caregiver leaves or returns
- Losing previously learnt skills (saying words like "mama" and "baba")

2-year-old

- Not using two-word phrases ("go away", "don't want", "go out")
- Not knowing what to do with common objects (toothbrush, mobile phone, fork)
- Not able to imitate actions and words
- Not able to follow simple instructions ("give", "come here")
- Not able to walk steadily and confidently
- Losing previously learnt skills (taking off shoes and pants, losing ability to talk)

3-year-old

- Falling down frequently when running, difficulty climbing stairs
- Drooling frequently, or having very unclear speech

- Unable to work out how to play with simple toys (shape sorters, simple puzzles, handle turners)
- Unable to speak in sentences
- Cannot understand simple instructions
- Does not engage in pretend play or make-believe activities
- Does not want to play with other children or with toys
- Does not make eye contact
- Loses previously learnt skills

4-year-old

- Cannot jump in place
- Problem scribbling using crayons
- Not interested in interactive or make-believe activities
- Ignores other children or doesn't respond to people other than care-givers and family members
- Refuses to dress, use the toilet or sleep
- Unable to retell a favourite story
- Unable to follow three-part commands
- Does not understand the meaning of "same" and "different"
- Reverses the use of "me" and "you"
- Speaks unclearly
- Loses previously learnt skills

5-year-old

- Only shows a limited range of emotions
- Swings in emotions (from shyness and sadness, to extreme anger, temper tantrums, and being highly aggressive, as well as unusually fearful)
- Displays prolonged periods of isolation; inactive, and withdrawn
- Is easily distracted, cannot focus on one activity for more than five minutes
- Does not respond to other people, or only responds perfunctorily
- Cannot distinguish reality from make-believe
- Can only play with a very limited games and activities
- Unable to give their first and last name
- Does not know how to use plurals or past tense properly

- Does not talk about daily activities or experiences
- Unable to draw pictures, just scribbles haphazardly
- Cannot use a toothbrush, wash and dry hands, or get undressed without help
- Loses previously learnt skills

It may be necessary to seek medical advice if these red flags crop up while observing the child.

Conclusions

The toddler can be delightful to look after, but they can sometimes be very trying. They are starting to show their independence, and they are learning how to manipulate the caregivers to get what they desire, and they really show their displeasure when they fail to get what they want. Scream!

Caregivers have to be consistently loving and sympathetic. Some toddlers can take an inordinately long time to finish their meal, and the caregiver becomes increasingly impatient. They can speak sternly to the child, but should not use physical punishment to force their intention. Many parents use the technique of "reward or consequences". If the child does what they are told, for example, they may get a simple reward like going out for a walk. But if they disobey, then maybe, they do not get to engage in their favourite activity. The types of rewards and consequences can be fine-tuned for each child's personality or situation.

The 18-month-old to the 5-year-old period is an extremely important phase of a child's development. Every opportunity must be taken to interact and educate them by talking and playing with them. Most paediatricians advise encouraging children to read paper books, write and draw on paper, and play with physical as opposed to virtual toys (real dolls, toy animals, BLOCKS, modelling arts and crafts, musical instruments, pretend cooking, building castles, etc). Physical activities like sports, dance, cycling, and running, are all very important for the child's development. Variety is the spice of life.

These days, toddlers are sent to preschool at an increasingly younger age, and parents start giving them music, art, and language lessons very early. There are pros and cons for starting so young. Kids are exposed to a different environments and to different groups of children. They can learn to socialise sooner and they become independent faster. Some teachers are good at detecting developmental and learning difficulties at an earlier age, which can lead to prompt intervention and therapy. However, if tuition continues and expands into school subjects, the child's life quickly becomes overcrowded and pressurized. Some may even be turned off by being forced into subjects they do not enjoy. Give the child some time to relax and play. Life is a balance.

Over the centuries, toddlers and their families have had to face many difficulties. It is a battle that every age has to confront and overcome. The worry with the current COVID-19 pandemic is that children are exposed to the virus, which may have unforeseen consequences. We need to think of novel solutions to achieve our goals of raising children who are intelligent, creative, critical thinkers, kind, thoughtful, have total integrity, etc. Everybody has a role to play, including parents, relatives, friends, teachers, health professionals, and others. The results of parenting and teaching may not show up for decades. But it is a journey every family must take.

References

1. MedlinePlus Toddler Development: https://medlineplus.gov/toddlerdevelopment.html
2. Raising Children. Child development: the first five years. Raising Children Network (Australia) Limited 2020. https://raisingchildren.net.au/toddlers/development
3. Centers for Disease Control and Prevention. CDC's Developmental milestones. Centers for Disease Control and Prevention 2022. https://www.cdc.gov/ncbddd/actearly/milestones/index.html

3 Intelligence

Introduction

I am sure we all know of friends whom we consider highly intelligent but who do surprisingly badly in school exams. And we also know of the opposite, where classmates whose intelligence we rate as below par, yet manage to excel at school exams. Some of these friends may even have taken an IQ test confirming their intelligence level, and surprise us by performing unexpectedly not only in exams, but also in their future careers. Are these just the exceptions? Let us try to understand what intelligence is, what the limitations of IQ tests are, and how our embracing of the tests affects our education system.

What is intelligence?[1,2]

Intelligence is a mental quality that includes the ability to derive and store information, the capability of learning from experience, the skill of adapting to and manipulating the environment, as well as possessing the ability to understand and handle abstract concepts, solve problems, think critically and creatively.

How is it measured?

In the early 1900s, the French government asked Alfred Binet (1857–1911) to devise a test to identify children who were struggling at school so that they could be given extra help. Together with his colleague Theodore Simon, Binet developed the very first intelligence test which was introduced in 1905.[3]

In 1916, Lewis Terman, who was Professor of Psychology at Stanford University, revised Alfred Binet's test and renamed it the Stanford-Binet intelligence quotient or IQ. He adopted and popularized the formula for intelligence quotient (IQ), which takes the mental age and divides it by the chronological age, then multiply by 100.[4] Mental age is obtained from a population study showing the average age of a person achieving that particular score. If your chronological age is 10 years, but your mental age is 13, then your IQ is 130. Conversely if you are 10 years old but your mental age is seven years, then your IQ is 70.

The first mass testing of IQ was done in 1917 with 1.7 million American soldiers fighting in the first world war. The soldiers were graded A to E, and those with grade A were trained to become officers. This was so successful that the armed forces decided to adopt the IQ test for officer training and selection. Lewis Terman then pressed for it to be used in schools, to improve their efficiency. In 1921, Lewis Terman initiated a long-term study on gifted children whose IQ was 135 or above, and were in the top 1 percent of his cohort.[5]

Epidemiologists plotted the IQ scores on a graph and found that it adopted the shape of a bell; hence the term "bell curve". Statisticians then arbitrarily took plus and minus two standard deviations from the mean (which is 100), noted that this corresponded to an IQ ranging from 70 to 130, and called this the "normal" range. Below 70, one is considered to have a low IQ, and above 130, a high IQ.

The "g" factor[6,7]

In 1904, Charles Spearman (1863–1945) noted that mental ability tests that measured spatial, numerical, mechanical, and verbal abilities contained a general factor or "g" factor that pervades throughout these different performances, and correlated with them positively. He proposed that there was a general intelligence that was shared among all cognitive intelligence tests.

This "g" factor has also been found to exert its influence in later studies, such as Howard Gardener's Multiple Intelligences, and Daniel Goleman's Emotional Intelligence.

Fluid and crystallized intelligence[8]

Raymond Cattell (1905–1998), a student of Charles Spearman, rejected his unitary model, and postulated that the "g" factor can be subdivided into two subtypes of intelligence, which he named fluid intelligence and crystallized intelligence (1963). Fluid intelligence is the ability to absorb, store and organise new facts in the head, whereas crystallized intelligence is the ability to memorise and recall factual knowledge. Both types of intelligences are required for success in life.

Three stratum theory[9]

In 1993, John Carroll (1916–2003) took Charles Spearman's general intelligence model, added one further layer, and called it the "Three Stratum Theory".

- **Stratum 1:** Primary Mental Aptitudes: Intelligence is made of individual components, such as discriminating speech sounds, handling basic numbers and simple visual images, spelling, formulating basic ideas, reaction time.
- **Stratum 2:** Complex Factors: Ability to handle broader factors, such as joining sounds into complex words and sentences, complex mathematics, moving pictures.
- **Stratum 3:** General Intelligence (g Factor): The most refined and highest level of intelligence required for learning difficult concepts, and its contribution to creativity. It combines all the abilities of Stratum 1 and Stratum 2.

Triarchic theory[10]

This theory differs from the Three Stratum Theory in that it focuses more on the way the brain learns how to produce intelligent or creative thoughts. The Triarchic Theory was proposed in 2003 by Robert Sternberg (b 1949) stating that intelligence has three main components.

(a) **Analytic Intelligence ("book smart"):** Some people are very fast in learning and memorising information. They study hard, solve problems quickly, and they do well in exams. This ability for the brain to assimilate, interpret and use information to solve problems enables them to achieve high IQ scores.

(b) **Practical Intelligence ("experience"):** This is the ability to use skills and knowledge learnt from our experiences, and apply them to everyday problems. To solve such problems, it would be important to know the culture, history, and environmental factors that can influence the process. For example, learning how to cook, do gardening, or riding a bicycle are learnt more readily by some people with practical intelligence.

(c) **Creative Intelligence ("street smart"):** The ability to adapt one's knowledge to solve problems in new situations. Inventing new devices, writing original computer programmes, creating art and music, getting along with people and avoid antagonising them, are some examples of being street smart.

Multiple intelligences[11,12]

In 1983, Howard Gardner (b1943) proposed the theory of Multiple Intelligences, splitting up intelligences into several components. He claimed that conventional IQ tests only tested linguistic and mathematical cognitive abilities. Several areas not tested were added to his list of multiple intelligences:

- Musical-rhythmic
- Visual-spatial
- Linguistic
- Mathematical
- Interpersonal
- Intrapersonal
- Existential
- Naturalistic
- Bodily-kinaesthetic

Gardener's theory influenced educational psychology by widening the definition of intelligence to more than merely linguistic and mathematical abilities. Many educationalists and parents realise there are many other areas that children can excel in, including music, art, dance, athletics, and social interactions.

However, there are many critics of multiple intelligences. One such critic is Jordan Peterson, who described it as "rubbish"! He claimed that the multiple intelligences were just different types of talents, not intelligence. It boils down to how you define intelligence. Peterson defines it as "the estimate of one's ability to succeed in hierarchies that are dependent on the ability to manipulate complex sets of information". Hence, music, art, dance, etc, are not included in this definition. The question is, should one take a narrow or a broader view of intelligence?

Emotional intelligence[13]

Emotional intelligence (EQ) is touted to be even more important than traditional IQ. In 1995, Daniel Goleman popularised this concept. People with emotional intelligence are not only able to perceive, understand and manage their own emotions, but they can also discern those of other people, and can use this ability to guide their interpersonal interactions.

Critics of emotional intelligence say that it is poorly defined and not easily measurable, and that its importance is overblown.

Social intelligence[14,15]

Edward Thorndike (1874–1949) described social intelligence (SQ) as the ability to understand and manage other people of all ages, genders, races, religions, beliefs, etc, and to act wisely in human relations. Social intelligence is measured through a series of questions and answers. E.g.: Discuss how you would handle the following scenario: An employee is always late for work, has low work output, and indeed has not delivered any results for the past month, and is now on the verge of dismissal. Candidates are assessed on their ability to discuss the problem, express different points of view, and suggest how to manage this situation.

Is IQ genetically inheritable?[16,17]

We have observed that high IQ students tend to come from high IQ families, often parents who are professionals. Of course, such families also tend to be wealthier, and so we wonder which has a stronger influence: nature or nurture?

To answer this question, there have been studies on identical twins reared together and apart, and these are compared to non-identical twins. Identical twins brought up separately still maintain similar IQ scores of over 70 per cent, compared to fraternal twins raised together (60 per cent) or apart (40 per cent). Adopted siblings with no shared genes raised together only have an IQ correlation of around 30 per cent.

The fact that identical twins have a 70 per cent correlation of intelligence means that genes play an important role, but because it is not 100 percent correlation, environment must therefore also play a significant role.

How good are IQ tests?[18,19]

The concept of intelligence has evolved over the past century; we have since expanded our definition of intelligence and have started viewing intelligence from different perspectives. However, the IQ tests themselves have remained relatively static. There are many tests available, including the Stanford-Binet we talked about earlier, as well as other popular tests such as the Wechsler scales.

If it is the first time you are doing IQ tests, the unfamiliarity may set you back. But if you have been practising these tests, you will have an advantage over the first-timers. Those unfamiliar with the language used to administer the test will be at a disadvantage. In addition, coming from a different cultural or educational background, having an underlying condition like autism, ADHD, visual impairment, or feeling tired, ill, or depressed, can all have an impact and lower one's score.

IQ tests measure the speed at which you solve mathematical problems, the ability to analyse visual and language input, as well as memory and information processing speed. Hence the faster you solve problems, the higher your IQ. Criticisms of IQ tests include the fact that there are many other capabilities not measured by conventional tests, including emotional and social intelligence and creativity.

Many special schools and classes aimed at intellectually challenged children require an IQ test as part of the assessment. The gifted program also has an IQ test for admission. Keeping in mind the limitations of conventional IQ tests, why are we still placing so much emphasis on them?

Can one improve intelligence through training?[20,21]

Until recently, the dogma was that IQ was static and unchangeable for most of one's life and could not be enhanced through training. However, recent studies have shown that indeed, IQ can be increased through repeated mental exercises. Several IQ tests involve vocabulary comprehension. By learning new and difficult words, their subtle nuances and the different categories they can be classified, one can score higher on IQ tests. Many parents and teachers give their children practice IQ tests, with the result that their kids have shown an improvement on IQ scores.

Is the current education system stratified according to intelligence?

The current education system, especially in Asia, is like a race. Students compete against one another through a series of tests with only the brightest emerging victorious at the finish line. There are a limited number of pots of gold at the end of the rainbow, meaning that only the top performers will be allowed to win. Competition is driven by parents and by society. The rewards of getting into top schools, university, top professions, are enormous. Elements of the IQ test can be found in many school tests, such as entry into the Gifted Education Programme, secondary schools, and universities. Ironically, to be accepted into special education schools for the intellectually challenged, an IQ test is often conducted. These tests are so ingrained in the establishment that it seems unlikely they will be removed any time soon. What is the solution?

Scholastic Aptitude Test (SAT)[22]

In 1926, several American universities decided to adopt the IQ test to standardise college admissions. They named their test the Scholastic Aptitude Test (SAT). Over the years, the SAT has evolved to be more than just an IQ test, and the name has also been changed to Scholastic Assessment Test (SAT) to reflect that. Only candidates who score above a level set by each individual tertiary institution will be admitted.

Modification or incorporating part of the IQ test has been used in many countries as part of the entry requirement to gain admission into educational establishments. Singapore, for example, has modified the IQ test and named it the Primary School Leaving Examination (PSLE) to determine the format of secondary education that is appropriate for 12-year-olds. There is also an IQ test conducted by the Singapore Ministry of Defence for boys entering National Service in their late teens. Many countries include an IQ assessment as part of their test for admission to tertiary education. For example, students applying to United Kingdom medical schools have to take either a University Clinical Aptitude Test (UCAT) or a BioMedical Admissions Test (BMAT), and international students applying for Australian medical schools have to take an International Student Admissions Test (ISAT). Embedded in these tests is an IQ component.

What is the average IQ of the top professions?[23]

Recent surveys show that the professions attracting those with the highest IQs are university professors, followed by doctors, lawyers, accountants, engineers, school teachers, business managers and administrators. Despite this, we know of successful entrepreneurs who have become extremely wealthy, but had to struggle with the education system as children when they failed exams, and they were even admonished by their teachers as being failures with no future ahead of them. It demonstrates a key point that failing book smart tests may not necessarily predict future achievements.

The Flynn Effect[24]

The Flynn Effect is the observation made by James Flynn (1934–2020) that over the course of the 20th century, IQ scores have risen by as much as 15 points. This is a significant and sustained increase involving both fluid and crystallized intelligence. The time-scale of the improvement is too short for it to be attributed to genetic causes. Proposed explanations of the Flynn Effect include better parenting, smaller family size, upgraded education, improved diet, and a more healthy population. The effect seems to be tapering off in some developed countries, while IQ continues to rise in developing nations.

What about intellectual disabilities[25]

Many special education schools rely on the IQ test for admission. An IQ of below 70 is generally the cut-off point. One of the advantages of attending special education schools is the significantly smaller class sizes that can enjoy a teacher-to-student ratio of between 1 in 3, and 1 in 12. This contrasts with mainstream schools where the teacher-to-student ratio ranges from 1 in 20 to 1 in 40. In addition, the teachers in special education schools are specially trained to provide a more individualised approach to education. Music, art, sports, and socialising form a greater part of the curriculum.

With current trends towards inclusive education, where barriers are removed so that children with disabilities attend the same school and the same class as their regular peers, this remains a challenge for the education system of many countries.

Conclusions

Intelligence is a most interesting and controversial subject influencing how we regard others. It is a good predictor of important life outcomes, including educational achievements, higher earning occupations, mental and physical health, and even one's mortality.

The IQ test has become embedded into the education system, and acts as a gatekeeper for entry into education at many levels. The test has served its purpose well over the past several decades. However, with the ever-changing educational landscape and the rising importance of original thinking and creative ideas, we need to change our mindset. How can we free ourselves from the iron grip of IQ tests?

References

1. Falck S. The psychology of intelligence. Routledge 2021. ISBN 9780367482930.
2. Deary IJ. Intelligence: a very short introduction. Oxford University Press 2020. ISBN 9780198796206.
3. Wikipedia. Alfred Binet. https://en.wikipedia.org/wiki/Alfred_Binet
4. Wikipedia. Lewis Terman. https://en.wikipedia.org/wiki/Lewis_Terman

5. Wilson J. What your IQ score doesn't tell you. CNN Health 2014. https://edition.cnn.com/2014/02/19/health/iq-score-meaning/index.html
6. Cherry K. What is general intelligence (g Factor)? VeryWell Mind 2021. https://www.verywellmind.com/what-is-general-intelligence-2795210
7. Wikipedia. g Factor. https://en.wikipedia.org/wiki/G_factor_(psychometrics)
8. Jaeggi SM et al. Improving fluid intelligence with training on working memory. Proceedings of the National Academy of Sciences of the United States of America 2008. https://www.pnas.org/content/105/19/6829
9. Wikipedia. Three-stratum theory. https://en.wikipedia.org/wiki/Three-stratum_theory
10. Vinney C. Understanding the triarchic theory of intelligence. ThoughtCo 2020. https://www.thoughtco.com/triarchic-theory-of-intelligence-4172497
11. Wikipedia. Theory of multiple intelligences. https://en.wikipedia.org/wiki/Theory_of_multiple_intelligences
12. University of the People. What is the multiple intelligences theory? University of the People. https://www.verywellmind.com/gardners-theory-of-multiple-intelligences-2795161
13. Cherry K. What is emotional intelligence? VeryWell Mind 2020. https://www.verywellmind.com/what-is-emotional-intelligence-2795423
14. Goleman, D. What is social intelligence? https://greatergood.berkeley.edu/article/item/what_is_social_intelligence
15. Wikipedia. Social Intelligence. https://en.wikipedia.org/wiki/Social_intelligence
16. Cherry K. Genetic and environmental influences on intelligence. VeryWell Mind 2021. https://www.verywellmind.com/what-factors-determine-intelligence-2795285
17. Plomin R & von Stumm S. The new genetics of inheritance. Nat Rev Genet 2018; 19: 148–159. https://www.ncbi.nlm.nih.gov/pmc/articles/PMC5985927/
18. Panfiloff E. Are IQ tests accurate? Enhancing Brain. https://enhancingbrain.com/are-iq-tests-accurate/
19. Robson D. Can high intelligence be a burden rather than a boon? BBC Future 2015. https://www.bbc.com/future/article/20150413-the-downsides-of-being-clever
20. Griffin T. How to improve your intelligence. WikiHow 2021. https://www.wikihow.com/Improve-Your-Intelligence
21. Kuszewski A. You Can Increase Your Intelligence: 5 Ways to Maximize Your Cognitive Potential. Scientific American 2011. https://blogs.scientificamerican.com/guest-blog/you-can-increase-your-intelligence-5-ways-to-maximize-your-cognitive-potential/

22. Ben. A brief history of the SAT and how it changes. Peterson's 2017. https://www.petersons.com/blog/a-brief-history-of-the-sat-and-how-it-changes/

23. Cherry K. Are people with high IQs more successful? VeryWell Mind 2022. https://www.verywellmind.com/are-people-with-high-iqs-more-successful-2795280

24. Wikipedia. Flynn Effect. https://en.wikipedia.org/wiki/Flynn_effect

25. Lyen KR. Intellectual disability. https://kenlyen.wordpress.com/2021/07/26/intellectual-disability/

Gifted intelligence

Introduction

"I brought my 6-year-old son to see you because his teacher says he has attention deficit hyperactivity disorder (ADHD)," an anxious mother told me. "He cannot sit still, keeps on interrupting the teacher by asking endless questions, and does not pay attention, reading books all the time." I asked the mother what her son was particularly interested in, and the boy immediately barged in saying he was interested in the ice tundra, astronomy, dinosaurs, and Harry Potter books. All the while, he was fidgeting in his chair, twirling round and round. His mother revealed that despite getting bad reports from his teachers, he always performed well in mathematics and other tests.

I referred him for formal psychological testing and the report concluded that this boy did not have ADHD, but rather he had gifted intelligence. His behaviour was overactive, not hyperactive, probably because he was able to learn things very quickly, and got bored in class when lessons dragged on at a snail's pace.

What is gifted intelligence?[1-4]

There are many adjectives we use to describe intelligent people, such as "clever", "smart", "bright", "brainy", "scholarly". Some intelligent people are especially talented in certain areas, like mathematics, language, music, arts and sports. Does that mean there are many types of intelligences? What is the relationship between giftedness and intelligence? And how does giftedness differ from talent? First, let us try to define these concepts.

Intelligence

Intelligence can be defined as a general mental aptitude that involves several capabilities, including the abilities to reason, solve problems, think abstractly, plan ahead, learn from experience, understand and memorise complex ideas.

Intelligence can be measured by an Intelligence Quotient (IQ) test. However, this is limited to mathematical, visuospatial and language measurements, but it appears that there appears to be a general factor (g factor) which crosses into other assessments of intelligence (see below for IQ tests).

Due to the controversy both in defining intelligence as well as what IQ tests really measure, we shall use the IQ test scores on its own merits. The IQ score is a measurable entity and statistics can be used to analyse any correlations, so we will not probe the limitations of IQ tests.

Giftedness

Giftedness is a quality or attribute where a person displays exceptionally high achievement capabilities in areas of intellectual, creative, artistic, leadership, or in specific academic fields.

Children may be born with the potential of developing giftedness. In other words, there is a gifted genetic seed which can grow and flourish best when given the right nourishing environment.

Giftedness is usually linked to a high intelligence, with an IQ of roughly 130 or higher, found in around the top 2 per cent of the general population.

Talented

To be talented is to have the natural ability or skill to do something very well, often in the arts, sports, and more focused achievements.

Gifted vs talented

There is an overlap in the words gifted and talented, both describing a person's great natural abilities. The difference is the word gifted leans more towards shining in academic subjects like maths, science and language, and

Table 4-1. Differences between talented and gifted

Talented	Gifted
IQ between 115 to 130	IQ >130
10%–15% of the population	2% of the population
Knows the answers	Asks deep questions
Is interested	Is highly curious
Pays attention	Gets involved mentally and physically
Has good ideas	Has wild, silly ideas
Works hard	Plays around, yet tests well
Answers the questions	Questions the answers
Listens with interest	Shows strong feelings, opinions
6–8 repetitions for mastery	1–2 repetitions for mastery
Understands ideas	Constructs abstractions
Prefers peers	Prefers adults
Grasps the meaning	Draws inferences
Copies accurately	Creates new designs
Absorbs information	Manipulates information
Technician	Inventor
Pleased with own learning	Highly self-critical

is often related to a high IQ. In contrast, talented refers more to achieving outside traditional school subjects; talented individuals excel in the arts, music, dance, design, sports and other activities.

There are fewer gifted people in the general population. Talented individuals are very skilful and have brilliant abilities in many areas including dance, music, design, sports, writing, and the arts. Gifted people tend to think differently and some say that they can be more driven. The major differences between talented and gifted are listed in the table above:

IQ tests and the labelling of giftedness

Despite the limitations, the most objective test for diagnosing giftedness is the IQ intelligence test. The Stanford-Binet test was developed in 1917 by Lewis Terman, Professor of Psychology at Stanford University. It was modified from the original Binet-Simon test (1905), and remains the foundation of current IQ tests.

Since then, many more IQ tests have been developed. For children, the most popular is the Wechsler Intelligence Scale for Children.

For entry into many educational programmes, The IQ test forms an important component of the entrance exams into some secondary schools and universities (see Chapter 3 Intelligence).

Gifted education[5-8]

It has long been recognised that some gifted children have difficulties negotiating the conventional education system. Their minds are often racing ahead, but they are held back by their slower classmates. To help with·this problem, many countries offer education for gifted children on a voluntary basis.

In order to be admitted into such a programme, children have to take a special exam, which includes an IQ test.

In Singapore, children aged 9–10 years old take a special test. The top 1 per cent of that year's cohort are admitted to the Gifted Education Programme. IQ forms the major component of the selection criteria. Although the actual IQ might fluctuate from year to year, in general, the gifted programme selects children whose IQ score is greater than 135.

Table 4-2. Pros and cons of IQ test scores

Pros	Cons
Reveals hidden talents	Self-fulfilling prophecy
Standardised method of comparing children	Measures only processes needed for successful test performance
Excellent predictors of academic performance	Biased against some ethnic minorities
Valuable for children with disabilities	Poor predictors of real-life situations
Predicts future success in a wide variety of endeavours	Unconventional responses are often penalised
Preference is given to teaching gifted children	Measures achievement, not ability

There has been a lot of debate concerning gifted education. The first is the use of IQ tests for admission into the programme. The table above lists the pros and cons of using IQ tests to select students:

Interviewing children and parents who have been through gifted educational programmes, the general consensus is that the benefits of the gifted education system outweigh the risks of remaining in a regular mixed ability class. Most children enjoy the programme — they like to mix with children of similar intellect, being taught by teachers trained to handle gifted children, being stretched academically, and covering the curriculum to a greater depth. Many of these gifted children continue to do well right through university and their chosen future professions.

One of the recurring objections to the gifted education programme is that it creates a class of elites. One teenager in the gifted education programme was asked if she knew a child attending a normal class in her school, and she answered: "I do not mix with normal students!" To minimise this concern of superiority and elitism, many gifted education programmes try their best to integrate the children of all abilities to participate together in non-academic areas including art, music, drama, sports, and community service.

Some critics say that not all gifted children remain gifted throughout their lives. This criticism has been tackled by allowing gifted children to leave the gifted educational programme whenever they wish. To encourage gifted children to remain in the programme, the decision to enter is a joint one between the child and the parents.

Children develop skills at different rates, and this is referred to as asynchronous development. If a child is gifted in a narrow area, for example, being good in merely one of the academic subjects like language, mathematics or science, there may be some pressure by the parents to accelerate the learning in the area that the child excels in.

In the past, a few schools practised double promotion, where the promotion of a gifted child to a higher class was accelerated. This can potentially create some problems. A real life example is an 8-year-old child who has a mathematical ability of a 14-year-old. The student was promoted to a higher class consisting of older children. This individual had social and emotional difficulties mixing with the older peers. One possible solution to this problem is, instead of having double promotion, to organise individual tuition outside the classroom devoted to the academic area(s) appropriate for that child.

A flexible personalised education system is recommended. With technological advances, such as online learning, it is now possible to tailor the syllabus to the individual.

Multiple intelligences (see Chapter 3)

Another criticism of using conventional IQ tests for selecting students for the gifted education programme is that it assesses a relatively narrow range of abilities, namely mathematics, language, and visuospatial. Howard Gardner proposed the concept of multiple intelligences in 1983, suggesting that there are other abilities like excelling in music, art, body movements, social skills, and others, which are equally important.

The idea of multiple intelligences has made us look at education more holistically. Perhaps we should view gifted children excelling in areas other than scoring well in traditional IQ tests. Maybe we should look for those who are good in sports, acting, dance, cinematography, and other areas, and give them the opportunity to develop these areas further.

Problems of gifted children[9–14]

Parents seek medical or psychological consultation for their gifted child because they might develop some challenges related or arising from their giftedness. These problems can arise not only in gifted students attending non-gifted classes, but also in those going to gifted classes. That means the problems listed below can coexist with gifted individuals; and the problems include:

(a) **Attention Deficit Hyperactivity Disorder (ADHD)**
    The 6-year-old boy described in the opening paragraph is one such example. The psychologist did a formal assessment, and found that he did not have ADHD, but instead, he was gifted. His restless behaviour, failure to pay attention, and his constant interruption of the teacher, is attributed to his amazingly fast ability to learn. The teacher caters to the average student, and spends a longer time repeating the lesson, which bores the gifted student.

(b) Disruptive Behaviour and Poor Social Skills

Some gifted children get so fed up with the slow pace of the teaching that they engage in other activities, like chatting with their neighbours. Others are perfectionists and when they hear their teachers or classmates say something incorrect, they will interrupt and correct them. Some gifted children have poor social skills and do not know how to interact with their peers. They may be perceived by their classmates to be egoistical or arrogant, and this can lead to arguments, fights, and being ostracized.

(c) Depression

Depression and suicides are found in gifted children, but it is controversial whether or not it is more frequent in gifted children compared to their age-matched non-gifted peers. It has been suggested that gifted children are more prone to depression and suicide because they have heightened sensitivities, as they tend to be introverted, overachieving perfectionists, or they become extremely worried if they do not fulfil their self-imposed high standards, and they may be prone to bullying by their non-gifted peers.

(d) Twice-Exceptional

The term twice-exceptional refers to a person who is both gifted as well as being disabled. For example, it may be a person who has a very high IQ and is also autistic. The area of special needs may be a learning disability, dyslexia, attention deficit hyperactivity disorder, visual or hearing impairment, or motor deficits. If their accompanying disability is missed or ignored, these talented children may be under a lot of pressure, lose motivation and therefore under-achieve.

Is there a male-female difference in higher IQ scores?[15]

The quick answer is no, there is no difference in the mean scores of male and females. However, it has been noted that females tend to do better in verbal abilities, and males do better in spatial abilities. The other interesting difference is that the variability in IQ scores is greater in males, hence they are over-represented in the two extreme ends of the IQ bell curve.

Does high IQ correlate with life's success?[16–18]

This fascinating question has been asked for over a century. Large-scale intelligence studies include Lewis Terman's Genetic Studies of Genius which started in 1921 and involved 1,528 children, and the Scottish Mental Surveys of 89,498 children initiated in 1932. Subsequently, there have been many more studies. Compared with people with lower IQ scores, those with higher scores are more likely to:

- Achieve higher education levels
- Hold more prestigious occupations (E.g. engineers, accountants, doctors, lawyers)
- Earn higher incomes

However, there are several unanswered questions and criticisms of these studies:

- How significant is the correlation between IQ test results and socioeconomic success?
- What about the contribution of other variables like the parental socioeconomic status or school and exam grades?

Terman's Termites[19–21]

Lewis Terman (1877–1956) was the founder of the Stanford-Binet IQ test, which was introduced in 1916. In 1921, he began a longitudinal genetic study of highly gifted children, which were later dubbed as "Terman's Termites". They were followed up until they reached 70 to 80 years of age. Altogether, he recruited 1,528 participants between the ages of 3 to 28, who had an IQ of >135, comprising 1 per cent of the general population, which he labelled "genius". There were 856 boys and 672 girls, mostly from California, and they were predominantly white and middle class. The finding was summarised as: "The gifted child becomes the gifted adult." His Termites had ten times the national rate of earning a university bachelor's degree of that era. A significant number of graduates went on to earn postgraduate degrees: 57 doctors, 92 lawyers, and 97 PhDs which were exceptional achievements for that time. The salaries of his Termites were also significantly higher than the matched median per capita income. They were more happily married, healthier, had lower crime rates, and lived longer. This achievement did not continue to the second generation.

It is of interest to note that two subjects rejected by Terman because their IQ fell below 135, went on to win a Nobel Prize each. Hence the joke suggesting that if you want to win a Nobel Prize, you should not have too high an IQ!

Lewis Terman recommended helping highly gifted children through special gifted education, trained teachers, as well as employing enriched and accelerated curriculum. The benefits of this approach has been vindicated by more recent studies in several other countries.

Selected examples of high IQ gifted individuals

Lady Gaga (b 1986)[22]

The evidence that Lady Gaga has a high IQ is based on the fact she was admitted into the summer programme Johns Hopkins University Center for Talented Youth which takes in the top 1 per cent in terms of IQ score. Although it does not prove she is in the top 1 per cent of IQ, the following achievements support this possibility: She won 12 Grammy Awards, 18 MTV Music Video Awards, 16 Guinness World Records, one Academy Award, two Golden Globe Awards, is one of the world's bestselling artists, and is an established philanthropist. Online posts estimated her IQ to be 166, but some will say it is probably not that high, and give her an IQ of about 135, which is still in the top 1 per cent.

Terence Tao (b 1975)[23]

He is currently regarded as the person having the highest IQ in the world. At present, he is Professor of Mathematics at the University of California, Los Angeles. He was a recipient of the 2006 Fields Medal, which is considered to be the mathematics equivalent of the Nobel Prize. He also won the 2014 Breakthrough Prize in Mathematics. In 2006, he was awarded the MacArthur Fellowship. Tao is the author or co-author of over three hundred research papers. He has won too many prizes to list here, and is widely regarded as one of the greatest living mathematicians.

Conclusions

Gifted children are valuable human resources for any country. If nurtured appropriately and allowed to reach their maximum potential, they can contribute to the future of their country and the world.

References

1. Wikipedia. Intellectual giftedness. https://en.wikipedia.org/wiki/Intellectual_giftedness
2. National Association for Gifted Children (USA). What is giftedness? National Association for Gifted Children (USA). https://www.nagc.org/resources-publications/resources/what-giftedness
3. Davidson Institute. What is giftedness? Davidson Institute 2021. https://www.davidsongifted.org/gifted-blog/what-is-giftedness/
4. Wai J. What a century of research reveals about gifted kids. Psychology Today 2017. https://www.psychologytoday.com/sg/blog/finding-the-next-einstein/201701/what-century-research-reveals-about-gifted-kids
5. Wikipedia. Gifted education. https://en.wikipedia.org/wiki/Gifted_education
6. Wikipedia. Gifted education programme (Singapore). https://en.wikipedia.org/wiki/Gifted_Education_Programme_(Singapore)
7. Ministry of Education Singapore. Gifted education programme. https://www.moe.gov.sg/programmes/gifted-education
8. Loveless B. Pros and cons of gifted learning programs in schools. Education Corner. https://www.educationcorner.com/gifted-education-pros-cons.html
9. Eren F *et al*. Emotional and behavioral characteristics of gifted children and their families. Archives of Neuropsychiatry 2018; 55: 105–112. https://www.ncbi.nlm.nih.gov/pmc/articles/PMC6060660/
10. Page JS. Challenges Faced by "Gifted Learners" in School and Beyond. Inquiries Journal 2010. http://www.inquiriesjournal.com/articles/330/challenges-faced-by-gifted-learners-in-school-and-beyond

11. Gaille B. 15 Intelligence testing pros and cons. BrandonGaille.com 2019. https://brandongaille.com/15-intelligence-testing-pros-and-cons/

12. Davidson Institute. Vulnerabilities of highly gifted children. Davidson Institute 1984. https://www.davidsongifted.org/gifted-blog/vulnerabilities-of-highly-gifted-children/

13. Gross MUM. Exceptionally gifted children: long-term outcomes. Journal for the Education of the Gifted 2006. https://www.researchgate.net/publication/234604339_Exceptionally_Gifted_Children_Long-Term_Outcomes_of_Academic_Acceleration_and_Nonacceleration

14. Transformations. Unexpected consequences of growing up gifted. Transformations 2020. https://www.mytransformations.com/post/unexpected-consequences-of-growing-up-gifted

15. Wikipedia. Sex differences in intelligence. https://en.wikipedia.org/wiki/Sex_differences_in_intelligence

16. Pumpkin Person. The incredible correlation between IQ and income. Pumpkin Person 2016. https://pumpkinperson.com/2016/02/11/the-incredible-correlation-between-iq-income/

17. Deary IJ et al. The impact of childhood intelligence on later life. Journal of Personality and Social Psychology 2004; 86: 130–147. https://www.researchgate.net/publication/289963900_The_Impact_of_Childhood_Intelligence_on_Later_Life_Following_Up_the_Scottish_Mental_Surveys_of_1932_and_1947

18. Lo CF. Is there a relationship between high IQ scores and positive life outcomes? Psychology 2017; 8: 627–635. https://file.scirp.org/pdf/PSYCH_2017032816410282.pdf

19. Leslie M. The vexing legacy of Lewis Terman. Stanford Magazine 2000. https://stanfordmag.org/contents/the-vexing-legacy-of-lewis-terman

20. Kaufman SB. The truth about the "termites". Psychology Today 2009. https://www.psychologytoday.com/sg/blog/beautiful-minds/200909/the-truth-about-the-termites

21. Cherry K. Are people with high IQs more successful? A modern look at Terman's study of the gifted. VeryWell Mind 2022. https://www.verywellmind.com/are-people-with-high-iqs-more-successful-2795280

22. Wikipedia. Lady Gaga. https://en.wikipedia.org/wiki/Lady_Gaga

23. Wikipedia. Terence Tao. https://en.wikipedia.org/wiki/Terence_Tao

5 Creativity

Introduction

One mother complained that her son's kindergarten teacher told him that he had coloured the sky wrongly, and that there was no such thing as a green sky. Another mother informed me her daughter had been criticised by her primary school teacher for asking too many questions: "Shut up and stop wasting everybody's time!" I could go on with more examples.

Is our education system too rigid? Is it doing enough to foster creative thinking?

Definition of creativity[1-3]

Creativity is the ability to generate new and imaginative ideas that can have potential value or help solve problems.

What are the benefits of creative thinking?

We take for granted the myriad of new ideas and inventions that have transformed our lives throughout human history. In science and technology, it ranges from the invention of the wheel, all the way to space travel. The same goes for biological ideas ranging from cultivating food to battling pandemics. In communication, we go from the invention of writing right up to the worldwide phenomenon that is the Internet. In the arts, we can express ourselves from paintings to 3D movies.

Measuring creativity[4,5]

How do we assess creativity? The most popular test is the Torrance Test of creative thinking (see below). Psychologist Robert Sternberg criticised current methods of assessing creativity, saying: "Creativity testing as it is now done is often based on a defective assumption that different kinds of creativity can be compressed into a single unidimensional scale." Trying to decide which ideas are more creative than others is also very subjective. However, despite their inaccuracy, creativity tests remain quite popular.

Torrance Test of creative thinking[6]

The Torrance Test is the most widely used test, and it evaluates divergent thinking and problem-solving skills. There is a verbal component where one has to guess the causes or consequences of a given scenario, list unusual uses of an object (e.g. a book), and imagine "just suppose..." ideas. There is also a visual test of creativity, where one is asked to draw something original when given marked cues or complete a picture when given only a curved line.

Genetics and neuroscience of creativity[7–11]

Creativity is one of the most complex of human neurological processes, yet it defies precise definitions and objective measurements. If we cannot accurately assess what creativity is, then any neuroscientific study will be subjected to challenge by critics. Broadly speaking, creativity most likely has a genetic and environmental aetiology. There are families of famous artists, music composers, writers, research scientists, and other creative professions, suggesting genetic influences. Studies of identical and fraternal twins have shown that there is a genetic component to creativity. Gene polymorphism studies have also shown that genes play a role in divergent thinking. But we cannot ignore the fact that environmental factors can also play an important role in creativity. Parents, teachers and mentors can certainly inspire an individual to explore creative activities.

Which part of the brain is involved in creativity? With such a multifaceted process as creativity, it would be expected that many parts of the brain are involved. No single area of the brain has been found to be responsible for creative thoughts. Indeed, multiple areas of the brain are engaged, and they join up and interact through networks to formulate new ideas. However, certain areas seem to be deployed more frequently.

Functional Magnetic Resonance Imaging (fMRI)[12,13]

Charles J Limb and colleagues conducted a number of studies on music improvisation and rappers spontaneously conceiving new words while their brain activities were recorded in real time by fMRI. He found that there was increased activity in the medial prefrontal cortex of the brain, an area responsible for stimulus-independent internal generation of ideas. He also found reduced dorsolateral prefrontal cortex activity, a part of the brain responsible for self-awareness. By decreasing activities in this part of the brain, one loses a sense of self, time and place, and enters a state of daydreaming, meditation or hypnosis. This removes the inhibition by the self-awareness filter and allows for a free flow of information.

Nicola De Pisapia and colleagues found equivalent fMRI activities and brain connections in professional visual artists. They concluded that creativity can be viewed as a careful balance between top-down executive control and more free-thinking mind-wandering processes.

These and other studies looking at brain activities and network connections in creative people help us explore the neurophysiology of creativity. Hopefully, this can enable us to discover how brain exercises, body training, diet, socialising, and the physical environment can boost creativity.

Electroencephalogram (EEG)[14]

The EEG of creative people have been studied, and those engaged in creative activities appear to activate alpha electrical brain waves. Alpha brain waves are usually associated with daydreaming, meditation, or practising mindfulness. Research suggests that this type of brain wave activity may reflect the reduction of depressive symptoms, and at the same time, correlate with an increase in creative thoughts.

How to stimulate creative thinking

There are many suggestions on how we can stimulate creative thinking. No one method is better or worse than another. Indeed, it is quite likely that creative people may employ several techniques to arrive at their own flash of genius.

(a) **Alex Osborn (1888–1966): Brainstorming**[15]

Alex Osborn is regarded as the father of brainstorming, an idea he launched in the book "How to Think Up", published in 1942. Brainstorming is a group activity where participants share ideas the moment they come to mind. It continues to be an important part of creativity, and nowadays during the COVID-19 pandemic, people can meet online to brainstorm even if they cannot interact face-to-face.

(b) **Joy Paul Guilford (1897–1987): Divergent vs Convergent Thinking**[16,17]

Divergent thinking is an approach where you try to generate as many different ideas as possible within a time limit. Some people break down a concept into its individual components so as to gain deeper understanding into the issue, while others prefer spontaneous free-flowing random generation of ideas. Once many ideas are engendered, one can then turn to convergent thinking. This means you do the opposite and try to weed out the ineffectual ideas by analytical critical thinking to select only the most useful ideas.

(c) **Edward de Bono (1933–2021): Lateral Thinking, Six Thinking Hats**[18]

In 1967, Edward de Bono promoted JP Guilford's divergent thinking in his book "Lateral Thinking", which employs indirect and creative approaches via reasoning that is not immediately obvious. In 1985, he published the book "The Six Thinking Hats" where he proposed six different ways of analysing a problem, using conflict-free parallel thinking processes. These six ways of viewing problems can help stimulate creative thinking:

* The red hat: The emotional heart hat, focusing on feelings and instinct
* The green hat: The creative hat, where ideas are abundant and critical comments few

* The blue hat: The conductor's hat, used for management and control
* The yellow hat: The optimistic hat, used to look for positive outcomes
* The white hat: The objective hat, which focuses on facts and logic
* The black hat: The judge's hat, that uses critical judgement to predict negative outcomes

(d) Tony Buzan (1942–2019): Mind Maps[19]

Tony Buzan popularised the concept of "Mind Maps" where one visualises one's thoughts by drawing a map of images to help understand how ideas relate to one another. This technique has been found to boost one's creativity because drawing concepts helps some people clarify their thinking and generate more ideas.

(e) Mihaly Csikszentmihalyi (b1934): The Flow[20,21]

Mihaly Csikszentmihalyi described The Flow in 1975 as "being completely involved in an activity for its own sake". One is so passionately focused on a singular idea that the individual is totally immersed and is oblivious of time and of themselves. This state of mind helps remove constraints on thinking, and during this period, some of the best creative ideas flow freely.

(f) Arne Dietrich (b1968): Predictive System[22]

Arne Dietrich emphasised the importance of the predictive aspect of neurological function which he placed as the foundation of creative thinking. All new ideas are influenced by older ideas. By challenging established orthodoxy, and reaching out to the future, imaginative original concepts can be generated. Dietrich also devised a matrix of the different types of creative thinking.

(g) Drew Boyd and Jacob Goldenberg: Thinking Inside the Box[23]

Going against the grain, Drew Boyd and Jacob Goldenberg argued that creative thinking is best expressed by using familiar existing concepts and juggling them around to churn out new ideas. This is counterintuitive and appears to be a potent and effective approach to creativity.

(h) Keith Sawyer (b1960): Stages of Creativity[24]

In 2013, Keith Sawyer suggested the eight stages of creativity, expanding on the earlier classification of four stages (Wallace, 1926). This compilation of the steps towards creativity may help some people plan and expand on the techniques employed to create new ideas.

What stimulates creativity?[25–28]

There are numerous suggestions in the media on how to improve one's creativity. Unfortunately, most of the recommendations are not based on scientific evidence. However, with the application of fMRI, positron emission tomography (PET) scans, and electroencephalography, there are newer publications providing objective evidence as to which advice can better enhance creativity.

Dreams and sleep[29,30]

Many studies have found greater creative brain activity during sleep, especially during rapid eye movement (REM) sleep, when a person is dreaming.

The people listed in the table below assert that dreams precipitated their ground-breaking ideas. But the effect of sleep on creativity is rather complicated. Studies have shown that insomnia may actually increase creativity in some people. Perhaps one possible explanation is that to benefit from REM sleep that generates creative thoughts, one needs to wake up in the middle of a dream. Insomnia might therefore help in this situation.

Table 5-1.   Famous works that originated from dreams

Creator	Creation
Albert Einstein	Theory of Relativity
Dmitry Mendeleyev	Periodic table
James Watson	DNA
Niels Bohr	Structure of the atom
Otto Loewi	Chemical neurotransmission
Friedrich August Kekulé	Benzene ring
Thomas Edison	Numerous inventions
Srinivasa Ramanujan	Mathematical theorems
Paul McCartney	Song "Yesterday"
Salvador Dali	Painting "Persistence of Memory"
Stephen King	Book "Dreamcatcher"

Creative personality[31]

We are now entering an area of unsupported scientific evidence, only our own personal anecdotes. If cracking jokes is a form of creativity, then obviously those individuals who have a good sense of humour are immediately labelled as creative. It has been observed that both introverts and extroverts can be creative. This makes the observation bizarre, since everybody belongs to one or other of these groups. However, there do seem to be some personality traits associated with creative persons. These include people who tend to daydream, are intensely curious, are quite eccentric, and are fiercely independent thinkers.

Should we herd all creative people into one pack of cards? Let us take music composers, artists, designers, choreographers, authors, poets, teachers, research scientists, inventors, entrepreneurs, computer programmers, digital creator, chefs, etc.: Are they all different? Or do they create alike? Are there different styles or modes of creativity?

Habits and personalities of creative people

Having worked with creative musicians, writers, painters, research scientists, computer programmers, chefs, etc., I realise that each individual is different. Some are very sociable and love meeting people while others are introverted and avoid socialising; some behave like children while others are very formal; some have a good sense of humour while others have none; some work assiduously and meet deadlines while other are procrastinators and often fail to complete their work on time. I have also not seen any differences in the ratio of creative males to females, no particular preponderance of any IQ level, ethnic groups or belief systems, nor any of their love preferences. In other words, there is a rainbow of habits and personality types among the creative community. They cover the whole of humanity.

Education and creativity[32–34]

The world is facing many major problems, including the COVID-19 pandemic, climate change, religious, economic and political wars, and people dying of disease, starvation and armed conflict. To solve these problems, we need to find new creative solutions. One of the fundamental ways of increasing the number of creative people is through education.

There are ample criticisms of the current education system, targeting many countries worldwide. They range from overloading students with too much factual information; shoving too many tests and exams down their metaphorical throats; comparing students with one another so that not only do students become over-competitive but so do their parents. In addition, the class sizes tend to be too large, resulting in poor interactions between teachers and students which gives rise to one-directional teaching. Many schools spoon-feed their students with redundant outdated facts; and some schools are unable to provide a good balance between the sciences, the arts, sports and social activities. Some schools start very early in the morning with the result that students are often half-asleep in class. There are many more criticisms. The bottom line is that if we are to solve the world's problems, we need new solutions, and that means our education system must find innovative ways to cultivate creative thinkers.

COVID-19 pandemic and creativity[35]

The COVID-19 pandemic has had good and bad effects on creativity. Theatres, live performances, art museums, education and travel have been severely restricted in many countries, and this has had a detrimental effect on the creative industries associated with these art forms. But the lockdown and working from home have also had some unexpected creative results.

New drugs and vaccines have been developed rapidly to cope with the COVID-19 pandemic, and there are new ways of testing for the virus quickly. Online teaching and arts performances have become more innovative, and online communications has increased dramatically. There has been a sharp rise in the number of postings on all social media platforms, while software has been developed to make it easier for the public to film and edit their videos just using their mobile phones.

Conclusions

Creativity is the key to solving many of mankind's problems. Of the numerous ways to promote creative thinking, perhaps the most important is changing the current arguably outmoded education system. We need to encourage original thinking by improving the environment to enable fresh ideas to blossom. Make our dreams a reality. Our future depends on it!

References

1. Glăveanu V. Creativity: A Very Short Introduction. Oxford University Press 2021. ISBN: 9780198842996.
2. Wikipedia. Creativity. https://en.wikipedia.org/wiki/Creativity
3. Runco MA & Pritzker SR. Encyclopedia of Creativity 3rd edition. Academic Press 2020.
4. Isenberg B. Standardized tests "narrow," don't assess creative skills, Sternberg contends. Because Hamilton 2015. https://www.hamilton.edu/news/story/standardized-tests-narrow-dont-assess-creative-skills-sternberg-contends
5. McMahon M. What are some criticisms of standardized tests? Infobloom 2022. https://www.infobloom.com/what-are-some-criticisms-of-standardized-tests.htm
6. TestingMom. Torrance Tests of creative thinking. TestingMom.com. https://www.testingmom.com/tests/torrance-test/
7. Cohen A. Is creativity in your DNA? Artsy 2019. https://www.artsy.net/article/artsy-editorial-creativity-dna
8. Han W et al. Genetic influences on creativity: an exploration of convergent and divergent thinking. Peer Journal 2018; 6: e5403. https://www.ncbi.nlm.nih.gov/pmc/articles/PMC6071619/
9. Manzano O & Ullen F. Genetic and environmental influences on the phenotypic associations between intelligence, personality, and creative achievement in the arts and sciences. Intelligence 2018; 69: 123–133. https://www.sciencedirect.com/science/article/pii/S0160289618300266
10. Beaty RE. The creative brain. Cerebrum 2020. https://www.ncbi.nlm.nih.gov/pmc/articles/PMC7075500/
11. Cavdarbasha D & Kurkzek J. Connecting the dots: your brain and creativity. Frontiers 2017. https://kids.frontiersin.org/articles/10.3389/frym.2017.00019
12. Limb CJ & Braun A. Neural substrates of spontaneous musical performance: An fMRI Study of Jazz Improvisation. PLOS ONE 2008. https://pubmed.ncbi.nlm.nih.gov/18301756/
13. Pisapia ND et al. Brain networks for visual creativity. Scientific Reports 2016; 6: 39185. https://www.nature.com/articles/srep39185
14. Fink A & Benedek M. EEG alpha power and creative ideation. Neuroscience and Biobehavioral Reviews 2014; 44: 111–123. https://www.ncbi.nlm.nih.gov/pmc/articles/PMC4020761/

15. Besant H. The journey of brainstorming. Journal of Transformative Innovation 2016. https://www.regent.edu/journal/journal-of-transformative-innovation/the-history-of-brainstorming-alex-osborn/

16. O'Byrne WI. Understanding key differences between divergent and convergent thinking. Wiobyrne 2017. https://wiobyrne.com/divergent-convergent/

17. Jules. Go beyond the basics of divergent and convergent thinking. Stormz 2021. https://stormz.me/en/blog/go-beyond-the-basics-of-divergent-and-convergent-thinking

18. Wikipedia. Edward de Bono. https://en.wikipedia.org/wiki/Edward_de_Bono

19. Wikipedia. Tony Buzan. https://en.wikipedia.org/wiki/Tony_Buzan

20. Wikipedia. Mihaly Csikszentmihalyi. https://en.wikipedia.org/wiki/Mihaly_Csikszentmihalyi

21. Miller KD. The psychology and theory behind flow. Positive Psychology 2021. https://positivepsychology.com/theory-psychology-flow/

22. Milne S. Arne Dietrich — various forms of creativity are governed by two different brain systems. Salzburg Global Seminar 2015. https://www.salzburgglobal.org/news/statements/article/arne-dietrich-various-forms-of-creativity-are-governed-by-two-different-brain-systems

23. Lassiter BS. Thinking inside the box. Performance Excellence Network 2019. https://www.performanceexcellencenetwork.org/pensights/thinking-inside-the-box-how-organizational-innovation-really-works-july-2019/

24. deBrabandere L et al. Zig-Zag and the art of strategic creativity. Boston Consulting Group (BCG) 2019. https://www.bcg.com/publications/2019/zig-zag-art-strategic-creativity

25. Berlin H. What time feels like when you're improvising. Awaken 2020. https://awaken.com/2020/09/what-time-feels-like-when-youre-improvising/

26. Barrett KC et al. Classical creativity. Science Direct 2020; 209: 116496. https://www.sciencedirect.com/science/article/pii/S1053811919310870

27. Dietrich A & Haider H. A neurocognitive framework for human creative thought. Frontiers in Psychology 2017. https://www.frontiersin.org/articles/10.3389/fpsyg.2016.02078/full

28. Larson J. What are alpha brain waves and why are they important? Healthline 2019. https://www.healthline.com/health/alpha-brain-waves#benefits

29. Wikipedia. Sleep and creativity. https://en.wikipedia.org/wiki/Sleep_and_creativity

30. Cai DJ et al. REM, not incubation, improves creativity by priming associated networks. Proceedings of the National Academy of Sciences of the United States of America 2009; 106: 10130–10134. https://www.ncbi.nlm.nih.gov/pmc/articles/PMC2700890/

31. Nesenoff A. The top ten personality traits of creative people. Tikvah Lake 2020. https://www.tikvahlake.com/blog/the-top-ten-personality-traits-of-creative-people/

32. Grigonis H. Can creativity be taught? The importance of creative education. CreativeLive 2018. https://www.creativelive.com/blog/creative-education-importance/

33. Elmansy R. 10 Tips to Achieve Creativity and Innovation in Education. Designorate 2015. https://www.designorate.com/creativity-innovation-in-education/

34. Shaheen R. Creativity and education. Creative Education 2010; 1: 166–169. https://files.eric.ed.gov/fulltext/ED521875.pdf

35. Mercier M et al. COVID-19: A boon or a bane for creativity? Frontiers in Psychology 2021. https://www.frontiersin.org/articles/10.3389/fpsyg.2020.601150/full

6 Memory

Introduction

"Wah, you have a good memory!" my student recently told me. "Sorry, but what's your name?" I asked the student, half seriously. I have no problem memorising biological names like dermatophagoides pteronyssinus, but when it comes to people's names like Sudjiatmi Notomihardjo, I am totally lost. Have you sometimes felt that you know the answer, but it's stuck at the tip of your tongue?

We will explore the incredulity of memory, as well as its fickleness. Understanding its amazing capabilities is still one of the major challenges facing mankind.

Definition[1]

Memory is the ability of the brain to encode and store information with the facility of recalling them later when required.

Without memory, it would be impossible to develop language, personal identity, social relationships, and using past events to plan future events. Hence, memory governs our lives.

Basic memory processes[2]

Sight, sound, touch, smell, taste and other sensations first need to be translated into signals that can travel along nerves. This encoding allows us to select a route on a map that can lead us to our memory destinations in the brain. The different sensations may stop by service stations en route inside the brain and undergo further processing before they reach the main memory banks. Once stored, we can periodically withdraw varying amounts of memories from these banks. Retrieval is an important step because the memories can be put to good use. If we merely store memories but never retrieve them, our memories will languish in the bank, like a dormant account.

Types of memory[2]

Memory can be divided into three major types: sensory, short-term, and long-term.

1. Sensory memory

The five major senses detect signals from light, sound, touch, smell and taste. They correspond to these five subdivisions of sensory memory: iconic, echoic, haptic, olfactory and gustatory. Sensory memory only lasts between a fraction of a second to at most only three seconds. It needs to be set apart and distinguished from "Short-Term Memory" which, despite its name, lasts longer (see below).

(a) **Iconic Memory (Visual)**
When a person is presented with an image or an alphabet for a fraction of a second, they are able to remember a few items for less than one second. These fleeting images are known as icons, and the visual branch of sensory memory is referred to as iconic memory.

(b) **Echoic Memory (Auditory)**
An individual can store a sound for two to three seconds to allow for processing. This auditory processing is known as echoic memory.

(c) **Haptic Memory (Tactile)**
When touched, the sensory cells located in the skin can store the memory briefly. There are many sensations, including light and heavy pressure, itch, pain, warmth. This memory is called haptic memory.

(d) **Olfactory Memory (Smell)**
Smells are detected in our nose, and the signals are referred to as olfactory memory.

(e) Gustatory Memory (Taste)

Taste buds in our tongue can detect food flavours, and are stored as gustatory memory.

2. Short-term memory

Short-term memory refers to the memory formed while you are paying attention to something, like hearing a brief conversation (Figure 6-1). This memory lasts between a few seconds and one minute, assuming you did not reinforce it by repeating or rehearsing the stimulus. Take, for example, a series of numbers or words like: Piano, Cat, Detergent, Quarantine, Cool, Pencil, Kiasu, etc. Then we ask you to write down as many words as you can. Most people can only remember around seven items, which is the reason why most telephone numbers (minus the area code) only consist of seven numbers.

This short-term memory is briefly stored in the prefrontal cortex (the front of the brain), and the signals are then sent to the hippocampus (deep in the brain near the ear). But unless it is processed further by the hippocampus, the memory only lasts under one minute, and then evaporates. In order to convert short-term to long-term memory, the sensory information has to be encoded by the hippocampus and then relayed to different parts of the brain for longer-term storage.

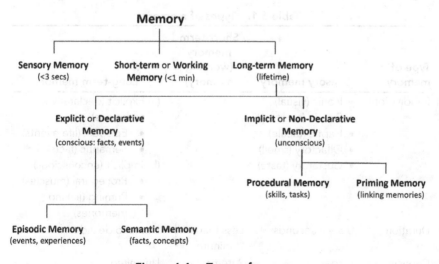

Figure 6-1. Types of memory

Working memory

Some people regard "working memory" as equivalent to short-term memory. But theorists nowadays regard them as two distinct types of memory. Working memory is also known as operative memory, and it is the transient storage of information while trying to manipulate temporary information (Figure 6-1).

Examples of working memory tasks include trying to add some numbers in your head, pattern recognition, or following a series of instructions you have just heard. The information needs to be held in your mind for a few seconds while the problem is being addressed. However, one may sometimes draw on long-term memory to resolve the issue. This is why working memory can differ from short-term memory.

Long-term memory

Long-term memory can be divided into "Explicit" and Implicit".

(a) Explicit Memory

Explicit memory is also known as declarative memory. It is defined as memories that you are conscious of. For example, you can remember

Table 6-1.   Types of memory

Type of memory	Sensory memory	Short-term memory (working memory)	Long-term memory

Subdivisions	• Iconic (visual)
	• Echoic (auditory)
	• Haptic (tactile)
	• Olfactory (smell)
	• Gustatory (taste)
			(a) Explicit (declarative, conscious)
			  • Episodic (life events)
			  • Semantic (facts)
			(b) Implicit (unconscious)
			  • Procedural (muscles)
			  • Priming (linking memories)

Duration	0.5 – 3 seconds	Less than one minute	Hours to decades
Capacity	Large	7 items	Unlimited

events in your childhood, like an accident you had many years ago. This is also placed in a subclassification called episodic memory. Another subdivision of explicit memory is known as semantic memory, and this refers to general knowledge facts, like the boiling point of water. Both episodic and semantic memories are conscious, which is why they come under the umbrella of explicit memory. These memories are processed by the hippocampus, then sent for storage in various parts of the brain.

(b) Implicit Memory

The other type of long-term memory is implicit (non-declarative or unconscious) memory. These are memories that you store unconsciously. The first subset of implicit memory is known as procedural memory. This usually involves your motor skills like riding a bicycle, driving a car, buttoning a shirt, or typing on a keyboard. These activities are performed automatically and do not require full consciousness.

A second subset of implicit memory is known as priming. For example, when you see a picture, hear a song, or smell something sweet, and suddenly the sensation triggers another memory, this is linking or priming a separate memory. Examples of this type of pairing are when you see a banana, you think of the colour yellow; or if you see a rat, you think of a cat. It is reminiscent of Pavlov's dogs that salivate in response to a bell.

Where are memories stored?

Short term memory is stored briefly in the prefrontal cortex in the front part of the brain. Long-term memory is largely processed by the hippocampus located in the temporal lobe found on the left or right side of the brain. However, not all long-term memory relies on the hippocampus; some are processed in the basal ganglia which is deeper down in the white matter, and the cerebellum, which is tucked away at the bottom and towards the back of the brain.

How do you convert short-term memory to long-term memory? First, you need to select eligible short-term memories, then you encode them into a format that can be stored for much longer period. But where are these long-term memories stored? This depends on the type of information. For example, touch sensations are conveyed and stored in the somatosensory cortex and the parietal lobe, both located in the middle of the brain. Emotional signals are relayed for storage in the limbic system which is found really deep down, near the bottom of the brain.

The hippocampus

The hippocampus acts like a gatekeeper and plays a central role in converting short-term to long-term memory. This sea-horse shaped structure is found in the temporal lobe on both sides of the brain, and all short-term memories are funnelled through here. More than just supplying an identification label for the short-term memory to wear, the hippocampus processes the information and directs them to the appropriate region of the brain for long-term storage.

Henry Molaison (1926–2008)

Probably the most famous patient that contributed to the understanding of memory was the late Henry Molaison, also known as HM. After a bicycle accident, he developed intractable epilepsy. The centre of the epilepsy was the hippocampus, so a neurosurgeon removed the medial aspect of the temporal lobe where the hippocampus is located. This resulted in HM losing his ability to form new information and as a result, fresh knowledge could not be remembered, a condition known as anterograde amnesia. However, most of his childhood and past memories were preserved, so he did not suffer significant memory loss of past events. In other words, he did not suffer retrograde amnesia. His working memory was also unaffected and he could do calculations. Also unaffected was his ability to learn new motor skills, which suggests that muscle memory is handled differently.

Lessons gained from HM include learning about the importance of the hippocampus in forming new long-term memories, and that implicit procedural or muscle memory does not involve the hippocampus.

Which parts of the brain are memories stored in?

Where exactly in the brain is long-term memory stored? Visual pictures are stored in the occipital cortex, with hearing stored in the auditory cortex

Table 6-2.   Where long-term memory is stored

Type of memory	Subdivisions	Part of the brain
Explicit (= Declarative or Conscious)	Episodic (experiences) Semantic (general knowledge)	Frontal lobe Temporal lobe
Implicit (= Non-Declarative or Unconscious)	Procedural (muscle skills) Priming (linking memories)	Motor cortex Cerebellum Basal ganglia Prefrontal cortex (conceptual) Occipital cortex (visual) Auditory cortex (hearing) Amygdala (emotional)

found in the temporal lobe on both sides of the brain. Concepts and ideas are stored in the prefrontal cortex in front of the brain. All the above input can engage multiple brain regions, not only the ones mentioned.

How is long-term memory stored?

Long-term memory can be stored from several hours to several decades. This is an incredible feat! How is this memory stored for so long? Much of the early understanding of the neurobiology of memory was through the work of Nobel Prize winner Eric Kandel, who studied the sea slug *Aplysia californica*. He used this mollusc because it only had one huge nerve axon where he could record its electrical activities after stimulating it either with a weak tactile stimulus or a painful electrical stimulus. This was following the exact protocol used for classical conditioning with natural stimuli in intact animals.

Use it or lose it!

When new memories are formed, the brain transmits signals from one neuron to another across a synapse. Experiments on the sea slug discovered the following: frequent usage of these nerve pathways will strengthen the synapse, but if unused, the connections are weakened and then lost; a principle popularly known as "Use it or lose it!" In addition to forming stronger synaptic connections, frequent usage of nerves will generate new branches or dendrites, which will in turn join up to form new connections. Both these actions are involved in the formation of long-term memories. The strength of a synapse is measured by the level of excitability of the post-synaptic neuron in response to a stimulus. Over time, high frequency and repeated stimulations can reinforce synaptic connections which will lead to long-term potentiation. As the name suggests, the resulting potentiated synapses can last a long time, and is the basis of long-term memory.

Memory over the life-span

(a) Babies

Why do we not remember anything below the age of about three years? After all, babies can remember faces, and how to manipulate toys, and point to body parts and pictures. Studies have shown that about 25 per cent of six-month-old babies can remember a sequence of events for up to 24 hours; they remember how to take off a mitten from a puppet's hand, shake the puppet's hand, and replace the mitten. Half the cohort of nine-month-olds can remember what to do one month later. And 100 per cent of 20-month-olds can remember how to perform a task one month after they were shown the task; and 50 per cent of them can still recall the sequence of events almost an entire year later. It is suggested that the infant brain is highly malleable, and that new dendrites form connections every day, and unused neurons are removed. This process slows down by the age of three years, and so adults cannot remember their experiences under 3 years old.

(b) Childhood and Adolescence

Over the next few years, children's memories steadily improve. They can remember the names of animals, sometimes even the names of the different Pokémon family members. From the age of three or four years upwards, many can do simple addition and subtraction, and read and write simple words. By the age of 10 years old, when they reach Primary 5 (5th grade), their long-term memory is quite powerful, and they can remind the adults what they have forgotten. When they enter the teenage years, their autobiographical memory can be quite strong and they can recount in detail the events they have experienced. Their prospective memory increases, so they are better able to remember and carry out an action that they have planned.

(c) **Late Teens and Adults**

Semantic memory, or the memory of facts, tend to stabilise in teenagers and young adults. Episodic memory, the recall of specific events in our lives, tend to slowly decline after the age of 20 years. We forget where we left our keys, whether or not we switched off the fan or lights, and what we were supposed to buy from the supermarket.

(d) **The Elderly**

Slowly but surely, memory fades with age. Past memories may be retained better but recalling new facts and new plans may suffer from lapses of memory. The incidence of dementia increases steadily with age.[6, 7] However, this does not mean that old age is a cause of memory loss: correlation does not mean causation.

Dementia

Dementia is a general term for the impaired ability to remember, but it also includes impairment of thinking, problem-solving, or making important decisions. The commonest type of dementia is Alzheimer Disease.

Amnesia

Amnesia is memory loss only. It differs from dementia which includes other manifestations, such as loss of some higher brain functions like reasoning abilities and making judgments. Amnesia can be divided into two major categories: retrograde and anterograde. Retrograde amnesia is forgetting past events, while anterograde amnesia is the inability to form new memories. The greatest correlation with amnesia is age, but as mentioned above, old age is not the cause. Of the known causes of memory loss, Alzheimer Disease is the commonest, followed by cardiovascular causes.[6,7] Anterograde amnesia is often the first to appear, followed by retrograde amnesia in most causes of memory loss. Pathologically, there is a loss of nerve cells associated with long-term memory storage.

Unforgettable[8,9]

The opposite of amnesia is hyperthymesia, a rare condition characterised by enhanced autobiographical episodic memory. These are people who cannot forget experiences in their own lives. According to Wikipedia: "Individuals with hyperthymesia can extensively recall the events of their lives, as well as public events that hold some personal significance to them. Those affected describe their memories as uncontrollable associations; when they encounter a date, they "see" a vivid depiction of that day in their heads without hesitation or conscious effort." Some people with post-traumatic stress disorder suffer from an inability to forget a traumatic incident that they may have experienced many years ago. Adverse effects include depression and anxiety, with some starting on drugs or drinking excessive alcohol.

False memories[10,11]

Also known as illusory memory, paramnesia and pseudomemory. False memory is a recollection that seems real in one's mind but is partly or wholly fabricated. An example of a false memory is believing you had submitted your homework but you did not; or thinking you had locked the door when you left home but you did not. This can be an issue when an eyewitness account is erroneously distorted and leads to a wrongful conviction.

The neurobiological basis of false memory formation may have several possible explanations. Perhaps the memory was improperly encoded, or maybe incorrectly stored, or wrongly retrieved. However, there is another possible mechanism responsible for creating false memories. This is based on the observation that the formation of memories is not purely the retrieval of stored old memories in its exact intact form. It has been shown that the formation of new functional connections is an important component of memory recall. This means that whatever we remember is actually a new configuration of neural network patterns, where we take bits and pieces of old memories, and rebuild them into a new final product. Thus memory is a reconstruction of old memories, and this memory is actually brand new. This process is prone to errors, resulting in false memories.

How to improve one's memory

The Internet abounds with advice on how to improve memory, or how to delay dementia. Some of the information is fake news, so one has to be careful what to believe. Proven methods include the following:

(a) **Physical Exercise**[12,13]

Physical activity, including aerobic exercises, has long-lasting benefits in improving memory. It improves blood flow, carries more oxygen to the brain, and protects brain cells by removing waste products. Brain-derived neurotrophic factor, a protein that promotes the growth of nerves and connects the new branches, is increased during exercise, which promotes brain plasticity within important cortical areas of the brain. Moderate to high intensity exercise also reduces beta amyloid plaques and tau-protein causing neurofibrillary tangles, all of which are believed to lead to Alzheimer Disease. Walking, cycling, and many "cardio" sports undertaken around four times a week for at least half an hour each time, will improve one's memory.

(b) **Socializing**

Meeting friends; joining social clubs, dance clubs, and choirs; going on hikes; playing mahjong, bridge, and other games; and having dinner together, can stimulate the mind and keep it active.

(c) **Exercise the Mind**[14]

There are several ways of exercising the mind, including doing crossword puzzles and sudoku; playing chess and mahjong; learning a new language; reading; and writing. All are effective in improving one's memory.

(d) **Sleep**[15,16]

The relationship between sleep and memory is complex. Sleep consolidates learning and allows information to be stored more efficiently. Lack of sleep impairs one's ability to focus and remember information as proficiently. Studies have shown that during sleep, some of the toxins that affect the brain are removed, and connections between nerves in the brain are strengthened, thus enhancing the building of memories.

(e) **Diet**[17]

There is a lot of advice advocating which foods to eat and which to avoid for memory enhancement. Your parents are right when they ask you to eat more vegetables. Fruits are also encouraged, especially apples, oranges, and berries. Omega-3 fatty acids found in salmon, mackerel, tuna, sardines, and flaxseed, walnuts, almonds, hazelnuts, peanuts, and gingko nuts are also recommended. The common denominator of dietary advice is that food which is beneficial for memory enhancement all contain substantial antioxidants that can remove free radicals that can damage cells throughout the body, including the brain. People who exhibit a gene called the APOE e4 gene are at greater risk of developing Alzheimer Disease, but when following the above recommended diet, their memory decline is slowed down.

(f) **Coffee and tea**[18]

Caffeine found in coffee and tea has a mild stimulant effect. Not only does caffeine enhance memory up to 24 hours after drinking, it has benefits in promoting long-term memory. Caffeine acts on nerve receptors known as adenosine receptors, and this transiently increases heart rate and blood pressure, but more importantly, it also promotes neural activity in the memory-forming hippocampus.

Imagining the future[19]

An important reason why memory is important is it can help us predict the future. Memories of the past are important in helping one to construct a vision of the future. Preventing memory decline in old age and sharpening our current memory are some of the greatest challenges facing mankind. Answers are slowly trickling in, and in the meantime, it is recommended that we engage in regular physical exercises, socialize more, exercise the mind, get adequate quality sleep, adopt a healthy diet, and drink some coffee or tea. Don't forget!

References

1. Wikipedia. Memory. https://en.wikipedia.org/wiki/Memory
2. Lumen. Memory. LumenCandela. https://courses.lumenlearning.com/wmopen-psychology/chapter/how-memory-functions/
3. Byrne JH Learning and memory. Neuroscience Online 2020. https://nba.uth.tmc.edu/neuroscience/m/s4/chapter07.html

4. Alila Medical Media. Long term potentiation and memory formation, animation. Alila Medical Media 2017. https://www.youtube.com/watch?v= 4Hm08ksPtMo

5. Busaz R. The neurobiological basis of memory formation. Psychopathology 2014. https://www.karger.com/Article/Fulltext/363702

6. Lyen KR. Dementia. https://kenlyen.wordpress.com/2021/07/06/dementia/

7. Lyen KR. Alzheimer disease. https://kenlyen.wordpress.com/2021/07/06/ alzheimer-disease/

8. Wikipedia. Hyperthymesia. https://en.wikipedia.org/wiki/Hyperthymesia

9. Lyen KR. Autistic savants. https://kenlyen.wordpress.com/2021/06/16/ autistic-savants/

10. Wikipedia. Deese-Roedinger-McDermott paradigm (false memory). https://en.wikipedia.org/wiki/Deese%E2%80%93Roediger%E2%80%93 McDermott_paradigm

11. Cherry K. False memories and how they form. VeryWell Mind 2021. https:// www.verywellmind.com/how-do-false-memories-form-2795349

12. Science Daily. Exercise improves memory, improves blood flow to the brain. Science Daily 2020. https://www.sciencedaily.com/releases/2020/05/ 200520084123.htm

13. Miranda M et al. Brain-Derived Neurotrophic Factor: A Key Molecule for Memory in the Healthy and the Pathological Brain. Frontiers in Cellular Neuroscience 2019. https://www.frontiersin.org/articles/10.3389/fncel.2019.00363/full

14. Karras T. Memory. National Geographic 2020. https://www.amazon.com/National-Geographic-Memory-Works-Improve/dp/1547854030

15. Rasch B & Born J. About sleep's role in memory. Physiological Reviews 2013. https://www.ncbi.nlm.nih.gov/pmc/articles/PMC3768102/

16. Wikipedia. Sleep and memory. https://en.wikipedia.org/wiki/Sleep_and_ memory

17. Mayo Clinic Health System staff. Maximize memory function with a nutrient-rich diet. Mayo Clinic 2020. https://www.mayoclinichealthsystem.org/hometown-health/speaking-of-health/maximize-memory-function-with-a-nutrient-rich-diet

18. Elfakhani M. 13 ways to get more antioxidants (and why you need to). The Conversation 2017. https://theconversation.com/13-ways-to-get-more-antioxidants-and-why-you-need-to-70035

19. Beck J. Imagining the future is just another form of memory. The Atlantic 2017. https://www.theatlantic.com/science/archive/2017/10/imagining-the-future-is-just-another-form-of-memory/542832/

7 Consciousness

Introduction

The greatest unsolved mystery facing mankind is understanding what consciousness is.

We think we know what consciousness is. We are enchanted by a beautiful sunset, inspired by heart-warming music, and lured by mouth-watering food. We know what's it like when we drift off during a boring lecture, drink too much alcohol, or descend into a food coma after a heavy meal. Consciousness plays an important part in our lives. Yet it remains one of life's greatest enigmas, one that we are still struggling to decipher.

In this chapter, we are taking a more elevated definition of consciousness; it is more than just differentiating wake from sleep, visual from auditory sensations, or how we control our behaviour. That is the "easy" problem of consciousness. We are using the term consciousness in its more sophisticated sense, where we are asking a deeper question: What do we really experience when we see colours, hear the sound of a violin, or feel the touch of our friend's hand? What exactly is this sensation, this feeling, this self-awareness? This is the "hard" problem of consciousness, and this is what we are going to discuss.

Definition[1]

Consciousness is the ability to experience and appreciate the world around us. This is achieved through our senses of sight, hearing, touch, smell, and taste. On top of that, we can use our brain to feel the rich palate of emotions whirling inside. Consciousness enables us to use our complex imaginations to think about concepts and ideas, and to plan for the future.

Should we exclude subconsciousness?[2]

Sigmund Freud (1856–1939) observed that even while awake, our minds are processing many activities that we are not consciously aware of, like being inside a room and forgetting the world outside. He named this intermediate stage between fully conscious and unconscious, the "subconscious".

If we are purists, then a definition of consciousness would ideally exclude the subconscious, because when subconscious, we are not fully aware of our experiences and sensations.

The unsolved problem of consciousness[3]

The major unsolved problem of consciousness is the mind-body problem. We can scientifically and rationally analyse how our sensations are linked to gross and molecular neuroanatomy, the neurophysiological pathways, the genetics, epigenetics, and the biochemical neurotransmissions of the brain. But knowing all the anatomy and physiology of the brain only tells us one side of the story. It does not explain how we actually feel what we feel.

The other half of the problem is referred to as the mind, by which we mean the subjective individual sensations, our experiences, our vibes, how we think logically, artistically, creatively and emotionally. In order to experience these feelings, we must be conscious. Therefore, a fundamental prerequisite of the mind half of the mind-body terrain is consciousness, including self-awareness or self-consciousness.

Over centuries, countless philosophers, neuroanatomists, neurophysiologists, geneticists, biochemists, religious thinkers, and mystics have all tried to solve the problem of how we feel, experience our surroundings, and be aware of ourselves. Their proposed solutions are still debated, and not fully resolved.

We shall examine some of their proposals and see the extent to which they have managed to solve the problem.

Descartes' Dualism[4]

René Descartes (1596–1650) tried to solve the mind-body problem by separating mind and body into two partitioned entities, a theory known as "dualism". According to Descartes, while the mind and body are separate, they remain interactive and can influence each other.

By separating mind from body, he had avoided answering the question of exactly how the two engaged with each other. We have known since time immemorial that when we die, the brain ceases to function. When we are brain dead, but our body is kept alive by a heart still pumping away, we can no longer have any subjective experiences. The reason is that in brain death, the structure and function of the brain cease to operate, and there is no way that our mind will continue to think or experience anything. The mind is dependent on the brain. Hence, Descartes' dualism is negated.

Mirror left brain: right brain theory[5]

A modification to Descartes' dualism is the split brain hypothesis. This proposes that each half of the brain exists semi-independently, and they are still connected to each other. Superficially, this sounds quite reasonable, since anatomically, our brain is already split into right and left halves. It was suggested that one half of the brain is responsible for the function of that half, but can peer across the chasm that separates the two halves, and check on the neighbouring half. Correspondingly, the other half of the brain does the same, and spies on the opposite side, and captures a different set of information. When combined, the two halves can integrate the information, and this creates self-awareness or consciousness. This theory does not demand that the division is necessarily confined to the left and right sides, and the two halves can be relocated anywhere. In fact, come to think of it, maybe there are more than two "halves" nosing around. This raises the complexity of the theory, and can be renamed the "multibrain theory of consciousness".

Do babies and foetuses have consciousness?[6]

Should we give foetuses and babies the benefit of the doubt and credit them with consciousness? As it is currently impossible to read the minds of others, and foetuses and babies are unable to talk and confirm whether or not they can have conscious experiences, we can leave this issue open.

The meta-problem[7,8]

In the movie The Matrix, Neo (played by Keanu Reeves) learns that the world he is living in is unreal, and that it is a world embedded in a larger reality. He has to decide whether or not to take the blue or the red pill: If he takes the blue pill, he can remain in the make-believe world of the Matrix, but if he takes the red pill, he would wake up and enter the real world. Well, he took the red pill and saved both the real and the unreal world. Philosophers David Chalmers and Andy Clark decided to explore this question: "Where does the mind stop and the rest of the world begin?" With technology today, the mobile phone and the Internet can be integrated into our mind and become our "extended mind". In essence, this is what Facebook's Mark Zuckerberg is alluding to when he called this expansion of our mental universe, the metaverse. This is the highly immersive universe where people everywhere can meet online to socialise, play and work. The real and the unreal merge and we may not always be able to separate the two. Our conscious real world is indistinguishable from the dream world of the unconscious.

Animal consciousness[9]

Do animals have consciousness? All of us who have owned pets realise that they can show love, happiness, sadness, anger and a whole range of emotions. Some pets can even communicate with their owners and persuade them to carry out the pet's orders. Are they conscious? Do they have self-awareness? We can employ the same argument for animals when we discussed whether foetuses and babies have consciousness. Namely, while it is possible and even plausible that our pets and farm animals may have some conscious thoughts, this cannot be proven indisputably. Therefore, we remain undecided.

A further question is whether the degree of consciousness depends on how high the animal is on the evolutionary tree, because it is generally assumed that animals higher up are more intelligent. Conversely, life forms lower down the evolutionary ladder, like insects, worms, plants, trees, bacteria, viruses, are less intelligent; are they then able to possess consciousness? If we are too liberal in our definition, then it is possible that atoms and subatomic particles may possess consciousness, a theory known as "panpsychism". This controversial topic is discussed below.

Can we build a conscious robot?[10]

Talking about intelligence, engineers are now able to build machines, computers, and robots with artificial intelligence. Some of these computers and robots are self-learning, and can even talk to humans and give intelligent answers. But do they possess consciousness? This is the million-dollar question. We will probably not know the stage at which the robot will become conscious, in the same way that we may never be able to tell if an infant or an animal has consciousness. The same goes for zombies. I sense that many of us humans will try to run away from answering this question, because we fear that one day, robots will take over running the world.

Panpsychism[11]

A rapidly expanding concept is that of panpsychism. First propounded by the ancient philosopher Plato, it was popularised by Bertrand Russell (1872–1970), when he suggested that we need to "think of the mind or a mind-like aspect as a fundamental and ubiquitous feature of reality". He suggested that "the mind ... exists throughout the universe". He named his theory "monism" to distinguish it from Descartes' dualism.

The word "mind" has more recently been substituted with "consciousness". This is interpreted to mean that elements of consciousness exist not only in all living creatures, plants, bacteria, viruses, but also in molecules and submolecular particles like quarks and bosons. When submolecular particles combine to form atoms, and the atoms combine to form molecules, and the molecules become life forms, the increasing complexity and interaction of the distinct "conscious" subunits collaborate and eventually produce consciousness and self-awareness.

This theory means that everything in the universe, the entire cosmos, possesses consciousness. It is only when the elements of consciousness merge correctly, that we exhibit a higher form of consciousness where we experiences the subtleties and nuanced feelings of our environment, and of our universe.

Panpsychism is currently considered a respectable theory, but it is not without its critics. Some people say that it is "just too weird to be true". They ask cynically whether it means that rocks, tables and chairs possess consciousness. Defenders would say that the weirdness of a theory is not evidence against it. Once again, we need to keep an open mind.

Integrated Information Theory[12]

There are many modifications and extensions of the panpsychism theory. One which is gaining popularity is the Integrated Information Theory (IIT) developed by neuroscientist Giulio Tonomi (b1960). IIT is the leading theory of consciousness today. It claims that information, by its very nature, has both a physical and mental dimension. When information becomes integrated inside a system, then an integrated consciousness unfolds.

The core of Tonomi's IIT theory states that when a system is conscious, it possesses a property called φ, or phi, which is a measure of the system's "integrated information". If you accept this theory, then do please welcome it with a "Hi-φ" greeting!

Tonomi and his colleagues have shown in volunteers that those areas of the brain like the frontal cortex that have greater neuronal connections have increased consciousness. However, Tonomi extends his theory beyond the brain, and predicts that every living cell, every electronic circuit, even a proton consisting of only three elementary particles, all possess some fragment of consciousness, albeit just a glimmer. Some supporters of the IIT theory also believe that the entire universe possesses a degree of consciousness.

Tonomi is not without his critics, but in his defence, he has demonstrated that his theory is testable. This might therefore open doors to medical and other applications to determine if consciousness exists, and how we can intervene.

Other theories of consciousness[13,14]

There are several other theories, including some that advocate a quantum hypothesis of consciousness. This proposal has been subdivided into sub-categories such as the holonomic brain theory of Karl Pribram and David

Bohm, and the Orch-OR theory of Stuart Hameroff and Roger Penrose. See the references below for more details.

The body

Let us briefly return to the body part of the mind-body problem. This is the "easier" half of the problem. Using modern technology, we have developed quite a detailed map of the brain and the subcellular structure of the neurons. Functional magnetic resonance imaging and positron emission tomography scans have given us real-time functional images of the brain as well as the neuronal connections present. Deep brain stimulation in a conscious subject has helped us focus on what the different parts of the brain can do and what the person thinks about when the brain is stimulated. We even have rather detailed knowledge of the biochemistry and biochemical reactions inside the brain cells. Recently, it has been suggested that the key chemical player in consciousness is the brain's dopamine[15]. Dopamine is a chemical released by nerves cells to send signals to other nerve cells, and by doing so it plays a major role in reward-motivated behaviours.

Mary's Room philosophical thought experiment[16]

Let us turn to the famous philosophical thought experiment, known as Mary's Room. I have modified the experiment slightly by making Mary totally blind from birth. However, she has a brilliant brain, and knows everything about vision from an objective physical perspective. She knows how light enters the eye, is detected by retinal cells, and she even knows how colour vision is perceived and differentiated by the blue, green and red retinal cones. She knows how the information is sent via the optic chiasm to the lateral geniculate nucleus of the brain, and that it reaches the visual cortex at the back of the brain, the occiput, and so on. But one day, by some miracle, Mary regains her eyesight, and she can see for the first time in her life. She can now see colours, shapes, movements, and is utterly amazed. It is completely different from what she had imagined sight to be. Despite knowing everything about the structure and function of the eye, the nerves, the visual pathways, and the biochemistry, she now enters the land of the sighted, and her view of the universe is wholly transformed.

As mentioned earlier, no matter how detailed our understanding of the physical aspects of the brain and its function is, we will not get nearer to understanding the subjective feeling of consciousness. We remain self-consciously blind, waiting for that flash of inspiration.[17,18]

Do you have a new theory?

Yes and no. I would like to propose two approaches using mirrors. The first is a theory — not an entirely new theory — but a theory that combines two previous theories.

The second is to borrow Snow White Queen's magic mirror. When the Queen asks, "Mirror, mirror on the wall", she gets an answer, "You are the fairest of them all". The mirror has the ability to read and assess beauty.

Part 1 mirror left brain: right brain

The first mirror theory is to combine the Mirror left brain: right brain theory with a fragment of the panpsychism theory (see above). But before I confuse everyone, I am not saying that I am referring to the right or the left sides of the brain; it could be any part of the brain. I am also not using the word "mirror" as a physical reflection, but as an interaction. The idea is that the brain is not merely one mirror, but maybe thousands of miniature mirrors that interact with one another. I also do not want to go down to the molecular or quantum physics depth of the brain. That rabbit hole is too deep. I stop at the neurons level. Hence I doubt that bacteria, viruses, and atoms possess consciousness.

The theory I am proposing is that when one neuron interacts with another, it starts a series of reactions. But it is only when a critical number of neurons interact with each other that this chain reaction erupts out of the subconscious. If it is the visual neurons that are stimulated, we can see; if it is the auditory neurons, we can hear; and if it is the tactile neurons, we can touch; etc. When the signals are sufficiently loud, it surfaces into our conscious thoughts.

I realise that detractors will attack the theory as making the same mistake as all the neurophysiologists and neurobiochemists in that nobody can really translate the objective into the subjective, the body into the mind.

And you may well be right. But in my defence, I think that my approach is slightly more pragmatic (more Singaporean), and does not need to assign consciousness to bacteria, viruses, atoms, and subatomic quanta. Most of the current theories engage subatomic particles like quarks and bosons, but I shy away from these elements.

Part 2 reading brain signals

The second part of my proposed solution to the Mind-Body Problem is to borrow the Magic Mirror and train it to read the circuits and electrical activities inside the brain. It will be like interpreting the electrical activities in your television set-top box. A highly intelligent computer (or Mirror) will one day be able to translate the TV signals into videos that can be displayed on the TV screen. When we invent a computer to read the comparable electrical-biochemical activities in our brain, we may one day translate them into visual, auditory, tactile, and other emotions. In other words, this means the machine can read someone else's mind and translate it into signals that another human can understand. So, the partial and tangential solution of the mind-body problem is to interpret electrical-biochemical signals into another medium so that a human can understand what's going on. By reading someone's mind with the aid of a machine, we are partially solving the mind-body problem. I read my own mind with the help of a machine. Hence I am self-aware, self-conscious. Voilà!

But if this approach fails, we may have to adopt Snow White Queen's technique... use magic!

Conclusions[19]

The leading unsolved mystery facing humanity is comprehending what consciousness is. Over centuries, many people have tried to solve this problem. In recent years, there has been a resurgence of interest, in part because of technological advances in exploring the brain. Like all scientific theories, some will survive the test of time while others will wither away. Hopefully, we are getting nearer to solving all the questions about what we mean by, and how we generate the different forms of consciousness.

References

1. Wikipedia. Consciousness. https://en.wikipedia.org/wiki/Consciousness
2. Longwill O. Conscious vs. subconscious mind. Medium.com 2019. https://medium.com/@ozgel/conscious-vs-subconscious-mind-do-you-really-know-the-difference-1196a2e05dc2
3. Jerath R & Beveridge C. Top mysteries of the mind: insights from the default space model of consciousness. Frontiers in Human Neuroscience 2018. https://www.frontiersin.org/articles/10.3389/fnhum.2018.00162/full
4. Wikipedia. Mind-body dualism. https://en.wikipedia.org/wiki/Mind%E2%80%93body_dualism
5. Higa K. The Roots Of Consciousness: We're Of 2 Minds. National Public Radio NPR 2017. https://www.npr.org/sections/health-shots/2017/06/15/532920899/the-roots-of-consciousness-were-of-two-minds
6. Lagercrantz H & Changeux J. The emergence of human consciousness: from fetal to neonatal life. Pediatric Research 2009; 65: 255–260. https://www.nature.com/articles/pr200950
7. Chatfield T. The man rethinking the definition of reality. BBC Future 2022. https://www.bbc.com/future/article/20220216-the-man-rethinking-the-definition-of-reality
8. Chalmers DJ. The meta-problem of consciousness. Journal of Consciousness Studies 2018; 25: 6–61.
9. Wikipedia. Animal consciousness. https://en.wikipedia.org/wiki/Animal_consciousness
10. Wikipedia. Artificial consciousness. https://en.wikipedia.org/wiki/Artificial_consciousness
11. Wikipedia. Panpsychism. https://en.wikipedia.org/wiki/Panpsychism
12. Wikipedia. Integrated Information Technology (IIT) https://en.wikipedia.org/wiki/Integrated_information_theory
13. Wikipedia. Holonomic brain theory. https://en.wikipedia.org/wiki/Holonomic_brain_theory
14. Wikipedia. Orchestrated objective reduction (Orch OR). https://en.wikipedia.org/wiki/Orchestrated_objective_reduction
15. Sahakian BJ et al. Consciousness: how the brain chemical 'dopamine' plays a key role — new research. The Conversation 2021. https://theconversation.com/consciousness-how-the-brain-chemical-dopamine-plays-a-key-role-new-research-165498
16. Wikipedia. Knowledge argument (Mary's Room). https://en.wikipedia.org/wiki/Knowledge_argument

17. Blackmore S. Consciousness, a very short introduction. Oxford University Press 2017. ISBN: 978-0198794738.
18. Scientific American Special Collector's Edition 2022. Secrets of the Mind. Scientific American 2022.
19. New Scientist Essential Guide No 12, 2022. Consciousness: understanding the ghost in the machine. ISSN: 2634-0151.

8 Sleep

Introduction

There is a debate being discussed in the news and on social media concerning how much sleep children need. In many Asian countries, children wake up at 6:00 am in order to reach school by 7:30 am. They are half-asleep during lessons, unable to imbibe very much information. This is compounded by the fact that many schools pile on a ton of homework, so children stay up late to complete their assignments. How much sleep do we need? What happens when we are robbed of our beauty sleep? We will explore the mysteries of sleep here.

Definition[1,2]

What is sleep? Sleep is a state of altered consciousness, with some inhibition of sensations, reduced voluntary muscle activity, and minimal interactions with the surrounding environment. It recurs in daily cycles.

What's the difference between sleep and unconsciousness?[3]

Both deal with loss of consciousness, so therefore there is some overlap between sleep and unconsciousness. The differences are that sleep is a normal natural process of transient slight loss of consciousness. A sleeping person will respond to loud noises and tactile stimulation. Unconsciousness is an abnormal state where a person is unaware of the environment, and is unable to respond to noise or other activities.

Another difference is that before becoming unconscious, a person may feel confused, disorientated, and then be in a stupor. In contrast, these manifestations of confusion and disorientation occur when waking up from sleep.

Historical aspects

The major advance in understanding sleep was the application of the electroencephalogram (EEG) on humans by German psychiatrist Hans Berger in 1929.[4] Electrodes placed on a person's scalp could record the electrical activities of the brain. This allows one to correlate electrical activities with the depth of sleep.

Rapid eye movement

Another landmark in understanding sleep was by Eugene Aserinsky when he placed electrodes adjacent to his 8-year-old son's eyes, as well as electrodes on other parts of the scalp.[5] When his son fell asleep, he noticed that the electrode pens tracking the eye movements were swinging back and forth rapidly. He announced this discovery in 1951, and termed it Rapid Eye Movement (REM) sleep.

Stages of sleep[6]

There used to be five stages of sleep, but in 2007, the American Academy of Sleep Medicine reduced it to four stages by merging stages 3 and 4. This resulted in three non-rapid eye movement (NREM) stages of sleep, and one REM, which is now positioned as stage 4. During all these stages of sleep, the person is relatively unconscious and is largely unaware of their surroundings.

(a) **Stage 1 NREM (dozing)** lasts 1 – 5 minutes
 Basically, this is the dozing off stage, the body has not fully relaxed, and there may be a few jerks or twitches. It is quite easy to wake the person up, and sometimes, they claim that they were never asleep although EEG confirms entry into this stage of sleep by showing theta

waves. If the individual is undisturbed, they can slip rapidly into stage 2 sleep after a couple of minutes.

(b) **Stage 2 NREM (light sleep)** lasts 10 – 60 minutes

Stage 2 sleep is characterised by the person becoming more subdued, with a drop in body temperature, muscle relaxation, slowing down of breathing and heart rate. The EEG shows sleep spindles and K waves. This stage lasts from 10 minutes to one hour.

(c) **Stage 3 NREM (deep or delta sleep)** lasts 20 – 40 minutes

This stage is referred to as deep sleep, because it is very hard to awaken the individual. Even loud noises and shaking the person may fail to wake them up. Muscle tone is completely relaxed, the respiratory and heart rates decrease to their slowest. The EEG shows delta waves, so sometimes, deep sleep is sometimes referred to as delta sleep. This stage takes up 25 per cent of the sleep cycle and is critical in restoring the mind that has been battered by stress and exhaustion. It also enables the body to recover and grow, and to fortify the immune system. Deep sleep contributes to long-term memory retention and recall. It is important for problem-solving and creative thinking. This stage of sleep lasts between 20 and 40 minutes. If one continues sleeping, this stage becomes shorter, and REM sleep gets progressively longer.

(d) **Stage 4 REM sleep**[7] lasts 10 – 60 minutes

During REM sleep, brain activities pick up to almost the same level as when awake. The EEG pattern resembles the woken state, but with additional sawtooth waves. Most voluntary muscles are immobilised, and some people actually become temporarily paralysed, unable to move their limbs. In contrast, the eye muscles move rapidly, breathing is faster and irregular, and the heart rate can increase with high variability. The EEG shows that the brain is very active in contrast to the voluntary muscles which are immobile. Hence, REM sleep is sometimes referred to as paradoxical sleep. Dreams are the hallmark of REM sleep. If you are woken up during REM sleep, it is more likely that you will be aware of your dreams. REM sleep takes up about 25 per cent of the sleep state in adults, and up to 50 per cent in children, and lasts between 45 and 60 minutes in children. The importance of REM sleep is that memories are consolidated, some recent memories are reactivated, and emotional memories are being stored. It is now believed that REM sleep is important in fostering creative thinking.

Dreams and nightmares[8]

"To sleep, perchance to dream" – Shakespeare's Hamlet

Dreams are hallucinations that can range from soothing to mysterious, fantastical and scary. Although dreams can occur at any stage of sleep, the most vivid dreams occur during REM sleep. Why do we dream? According to Sigmund Freud, dreams represent our unconscious thoughts and desires. They include repressed and unwanted emotions, experiences and aggressive impulses. By analysing dreams, Freud suggested that this enables one to access the unconscious and gain insights into the problems one is facing.

With the advent of EEG and other investigation techniques, some scientists believe that dreams are merely random chaotic firing of neurons, no doubt influenced by recent events and emotions, but devoid of any other significance. On the other hand, other neuropsychologists suggest that the purpose of dreams is to moderate extreme thoughts and fears, to reduce intense emotions, to help one adjust to the real world. In other words, it is like cleaning up the mind, sweeping away disorderly thoughts and hiding away terrifying nightmares and unhealthy desires. This is a neo-Freudian perspective.

Emotional healing, creativity[9,10]

On the positive side, dreams are found to have two benefits. First is emotional healing. In REM sleep, the stress molecule noradrenaline is quiescent. During this period, memory-related structures and emotions are reactivated because of the absence of noradrenaline. This enables the brain to process disturbing memories, calms them down, or tries to resolve unresolved conflicts in the mind.

The second benefit of REM dreaming is stimulating creativity. Many famous works were attributed by their creators to dreams that provided them with ideas that brought them their genius creations. It is during REM sleep that bizarre unorthodox images surface, and distant unrelated thoughts can get fused into an original breakthrough idea. The mechanism appears to be that during dreams, the neurons from distant parts of the brain interconnect in prodigious swathes. This allows for associations of previously unconnected parts of the brain.

Sleep apnoea[11,12]

Sleep apnoea is a sleeping disorder where the breathing stops repeatedly during sleep. Early warning signs of sleep apnoea include loud snoring, sudden awakening with spluttering or choking, frequent waking up from sleep, insomnia, daytime sleepiness or tiredness, irritability, forgetfulness, depression, anxiety, frequent night-time urination, and morning headaches.

Overweight persons, those with enlarged tonsils and adenoids, older males, a family history of sleep apnoea, alcohol or sedative consumption, smokers, as well as sufferers of nose allergies and heart failure, are more likely to develop sleep apnoea.

The main types of sleep apnoea are:

- Obstructive sleep apnoea, the more common form that occurs when throat muscles relax and the soft tissue at the back of the throat collapses during sleep.
- Central sleep apnoea, which occurs when the muscles controlling breathing fail to function. This can be due to brain damage following a stroke or infection, or it can be a neuromuscular disease such as amyotrophic lateral sclerosis.
- Complex sleep apnoea syndrome, also known as treatment-emergent central sleep apnoea, can be the combination of both obstructive sleep apnoea and central sleep apnoea.

The diagnosis is made by hooking one up to several pieces of equipment that monitor heart rate, breathing rate, brain EEG, arm and leg movements, and oxygen saturation during sleep. This is known as nocturnal polysomnography. The test is usually carried out in a clinic, hospital, or a special laboratory. A simplified test can be done at home, known as the Home Sleep Test where the heart rate, oxygen saturation, air flow and breathing patterns are recorded.

If undiagnosed or left untreated, sleep apnoea can cause hypertension, stroke, heart arrhythmias, heart failure, diabetes, and daytime sleepiness which can lead to increased accidents. Hence, the stopping of breathing while asleep is a serious medical problem.

Continuous positive airways pressure[13]

Treatment of sleep apnoea includes weight loss for obese individuals, quitting smoking, and medical treatment for nose allergies. Other treatments include wearing a mask that delivers continuous positive air pressure while asleep. One can wear a special oral appliance that keeps the throat open. If all these methods fail, then an otorhinolaryngology or Ear, Nose and Throat specialist may have to be consulted for surgery or radiofrequency ablation of tissues at the back of the throat.

Narcolepsy[14]

Narcolepsy is an abnormal condition in which an affected person sleeps excessively in the daytime, and can quite suddenly drop off to sleep. For example, a teacher in the middle of class dozes off unexpectedly. This is in contrast to students who frequently fall asleep because of boredom. Some narcoleptics may also experience sudden loss of muscle strength, which is known as cataplexy. There can sometimes be a family history of this condition, and uncommonly, there may be an underlying condition such as depression or drinking excess alcohol. The neuropeptide orexin, which stimulates wakefulness, is low in narcoleptic patients. The condition usually lasts the whole life, and the best approach is probably for the individual to take many short naps. There are some medicines that can be tried, including modafinil which inhibits dopamine reuptake, and methylphenidate, an amphetamine derivative stimulant.

Insomnia[15]

The opposite of narcolepsy is insomnia, where the individual has difficulty getting to sleep, or waking up prematurely. The lack of sleep can result in the individual feeling drained and tired the whole day, becoming depressed or irritable. Students suffering from insomnia will have difficulty focusing and learning. Insomnia can be due to chronic pain, drinking too much coffee, long term alcohol consumption, or psychological stress. It can also be due to a medical condition where the thyroid is producing too much thyroid hormone, known as thyrotoxicosis. Biochemically, people with insomnia may be producing excessive amounts of the steroid cortisol, or the stress hormones known as catecholamines. Brain metabolic activity as shown by increased glucose usage may be increased.

Non-medical treatments should be tried first, and these include regular exercises, meditation, yoga, breathing exercises, and biofeedback approaches. Medicines include sedatives like benzodiazepines. There is a new medicine available which blocks the arousal neuropeptide orexin.

Sleep talkers[16]

Talking in one's sleep is known as parasomnia, an abnormal behaviour that can take place in any stage of sleep, including stage 4 REM sleep, but more often in stage 3 delta wave sleep. For this reason, it is probably not a manifestation of vivid dreams. The words range from incomprehensible mumbling to long speeches, loud shouts and even swear words. Some sleep talkers appear to be talking to a friend which can be embarrassing to a spouse overhearing the conversation. Sleep talking is quite common occurring in about 25 per cent of young children, and less frequently in adults. They do not remember that they have been sleep talking, and certainly they do not remember what they have said. As it is quite harmless, no medical treatment is necessary.

Sleepwalkers[17]

Sleepwalking or somnambulism is an uncommon sleep disorder, more often found in children than adults. The person might sit up, open their eyes, and stare blankly, but do not seem to be aware of their surroundings. They can get out of bed, walk around, go downstairs, and sometimes go out of their home to walk in the street. They do not communicate with others, and have difficulty waking up when sleepwalking. They can return home and go back to bed, and have no recollection of their experience the following day.

Sleepwalking occurs during stage 3 deep sleep. If one parent has a history of sleepwalking, the chances of their child sleepwalking is 45 per cent. If both parents were sleepwalkers, the chances are 60 per cent. Many drugs have been used to prevent sleepwalking, but there is no convincing evidence that any of them are very effective.

The sleep cycle[18]

There is a sleep clock embedded in the brain behind the eyes, known as the suprachiasmatic nucleus located in the anterior hypothalamus right next to the branch point of the optic nerves. This clock is also known as the circadian pacemaker or the biological master clock. It is sensitive to light. The suprachiasmatic nucleus regulates the secretion of the hormone melatonin from the pineal gland, and this hormone helps one to sleep. The precise neurological mechanism is still not established. Melatonin is available as a tablet for those who are jetlagged, people who have daily work schedule changes (shift workers), and people who have difficulty establishing a day and night cycle. It also helps children who have problems with sleeping, and it enables them to sleep longer. The current recommendation is that melatonin should not be used for an extended period, because there may be potential long-term side effects.

How many hours of sleep does one need?[19,20]

Babies need 14 to 17 hours of sleep each day, but this gradually decreases as one gets older. For infants and preschoolers, they may divide their total

Table 8-1.   Recommended hours of sleep

From infants to adults	Age	Hours of sleep required
Newborns	Birth to 3 months	14 – 17 hours
Infants	4 – 11 months	12 – 16 hours
Toddlers	1 – 2 years	11 – 14 hours
Preschoolers	3 – 5 years	10 – 13 hours
Primary School	6 – 12 years	9 – 11 hours
Secondary School, Junior College	14 – 18 years	8 – 10 hours
University, Working Adults	19 – 60 years	7 – 9 hours
Seniors	>65 years	7 – 8 hours

daily sleep into smaller nap times. Toddlers need 11 – 14 hours of sleep each day, and many parents try to get their children aged three years and older to go to bed around 6:00 pm to 7:30 pm.

School hours

Many countries in Asia place a premium on academic excellence, and that creates a huge strain on children. Between the ages of 6 and 17 years, Asian school children may get up at 6:00 am because school starts at 7:30 am. Many are not fully awake yet, and they have difficulty focusing on the lessons. The syllabus is taxing, and they are often taught in a non-creative didactic manner. When the students return home in the afternoon, some are sent for extra tuition. After dinner, there is homework to do, and some extra studying. Most school children do not go to bed until after 9:00 pm. A 2021 survey showed that during the COVID-19 pandemic, Singapore school children slept only 6.8 hours per day, which is less the 7 hours slept in 2020. This is far short of the 8 to 10 hours recommended for secondary school children.[21] During the COVID-19 pandemic they may even stay up later watching TV, playing computer games or become addicted to TikTok, and many do not go to bed until past midnight.

During the more severe lockdown phase of the COVID-19 pandemic, there have been other effects on school children, including remaining at home for longer periods, watching some classroom teaching online, being deprived of face-to-face social interaction with their peers, and cutting down on sports. The deleterious effects of COVID-19 include a marked rise in depression and suicide rates.[22] All these psychological consequences can affect the duration and quality of sleep.

How to get a good night's sleep

No doubt, parents have different policies for their child and for themselves to optimise their sleep. For young children, we advise setting a regular bedtime routine for them to follow. After dinner, perhaps families can engage in some activities that their child enjoys. Limit watching TV or playing handphone or computer games. Avoid excessively strenuous exercises before sleep. When it is time for sleep, darken the bedroom and keep it cool with minimal distracting noises. Just before going to bed, it may be a good idea for the child to visit the bathroom.

Conclusions

We spend one third of our lives sleeping. We are slowly beginning to understand its value. Sleep is one of the most impactful undertaking we can accomplish every day to reset the health of our brain and body. It can help improve our memory, our creativity, reduce obesity, hypertension, diabetes and other medical problems. Ultimately, it will help us live longer and more healthily.[23]

References

1. Wilson S & Nutt D. Sleep Disorders. Oxford University Press 2013. ISBN-13: 9780199674558. https://oxfordmedicine.com/view/10.1093/med/9780199674558.001.0001/med-9780199674558

2. Wikipedia. Sleep. https://en.wikipedia.org/wiki/Sleep

3. Kayem M. How to tell if someone is unconscious or sleeping. WikiHow 2021. https://www.wikihow.com/Tell-if-Someone-Is-Unconscious-or-Sleeping

4. Ince R. The inventor of electroencephalography (EEG): Hans Berger (1873–1941). Child's Nervous System 2021. https://link.springer.com/article/10.1007/s00381-020-04564-z

5. Brown C. The stubborn scientist who unraveled a mystery of the night. Smithsonian Magazine 2003. https://www.smithsonianmag.com/science-nature/the-stubborn-scientist-who-unraveled-a-mystery-of-the-night-91514538/

6. Cherry K. The 4 stages of sleep. VeryWell Health 2021. https://www.verywellhealth.com/the-four-stages-of-sleep-2795920

7. Wikipedia. Rapid eye movement sleep. https://en.wikipedia.org/wiki/Rapid_eye_movement_sleep

8. Lumen. Dreams and dreaming. LumenCandela. https://courses.lumenlearning.com/waymaker-psychology/chapter/reading-dreams/

9. Yong E. A new theory linking sleep and creativity. The Atlantic 2018. https://www.theatlantic.com/science/archive/2018/05/sleep-creativity-theory/560399/

10. Mendelson WB. Sleep and Creativity. Psychology Today 2020. https://www.psychologytoday.com/us/blog/psychiatry-history/202010/sleep-and-creativity

11. Cleveland Clinic. Sleep apnea. Cleveland Clinic 2020. https://my.clevelandclinic.org/health/diseases/8718-sleep-apnea

12. Mayo Clinic Staff. Sleep apnea. Mayo Clinic 2020. https://www.mayoclinic.org/diseases-conditions/sleep-apnea/symptoms-causes/syc-20377631

13. Wang JJ et al. Continuous positive airway pressure for obstructive sleep apnea in children. Canadian Family Physician 2021; 67: 21–23. https://www.cfp.ca/content/67/1/21

14. Wikipedia. Narcolepsy. https://en.wikipedia.org/wiki/Narcolepsy

15. Suni E. Insomnia. Sleep Foundation 2022. https://www.sleepfoundation.org/insomnia

16. Suni E. Sleep talking. Sleep Foundation 2022. https://www.sleepfoundation.org/parasomnias/sleep-talking

17. Suni E. Sleepwalking. Sleep Foundation 2022. https://www.sleepfoundation.org/parasomnias/sleepwalking

18. National Institute of Neurological Disorders and Stroke. Brain Basics: Understanding sleep. National Institute of Neurological Disorders and Stroke 2019. https://www.ninds.nih.gov/Disorders/Patient-Caregiver-Education/Understanding-Sleep

19. Centers for Disease Control and Prevention. How much sleep do I need? Centers for Disease Control and Prevention 2017. https://www.cdc.gov/sleep/about_sleep/how_much_sleep.html

20. Mulberry Learning. Guide to naps for infants, toddlers, and preschoolers. Mulberry Learning. https://mulberrylearning.com/guide-to-naps-for-infants-toddlers-and-preschoolers

21. Khoo BK. Nearly 6 in 10 Singaporeans aren't sleeping well because of COVID-19, study confirms. CNA 2021. https://cnalifestyle.channelnewsasia.com/wellness/sleep-tips-insomnia-singapore-philips-global-survey-237866

22. Tham D. Suicide cases in Singapore highest in 8 years amid COVID-19 pandemic. CNA 2021. https://www.channelnewsasia.com/singapore/suicide-highest-record-elderly-mental-health-isolation-covid-19-1984716

23. Daniels PS. Sleep. National Geographic 2020. ISSN: 2160-7141 https://nationalgeographicbackissues.com/product/sleep-your-brain-body-and-a-better-nights-rest/

9 Bilingualism

Definitions

Bilingualism is the ability to express oneself with ease in two languages.

Multilingualism is the ability to communicate proficiently in several languages.

The skills involved in bilingualism and multilingualism include the ability to listen, comprehend, speak, read, and write in a language other than one's mother tongue.

Bilingualism[1-3]

It is safe to say that most people in the world are bilingual or multilingual, speaking two or more languages. Some countries place significant and important languages on their official national language platform. For example, India has 18 official languages recognised at the regional level, Zimbabwe has 16 while South Africa has 11 official languages.

Singapore has four official national languages: English, Mandarin Chinese, Malay and Tamil, and we believe that these are probably the most divergent languages in the world, as they do not share common evolutionary ancestries. On top of these official languages, we have observed that Chinese families often speak different dialects. These dialects can be so disparate that they almost qualify as a separate language. For example, a Mandarin speaker may not understand Hokkien, Cantonese or other Chinese dialects.

Nowadays, most schools teach a second or even a third language. Over recent decades, English has become a popular choice for a second language in those countries whose main language is not English.

Tackling bilingualism

Fundamentally, the brain tackles language in four ways. The first is the input when one listens to sounds, which is followed by the output of speaking. Then later, the input is reading visual images of words, and the fourth way is the output through writing.

The age at which someone starts to learn a second language can make a difference in the outcome. Let's take a hypothetical family of four who has immigrated to Singapore from a country where they speak a different language, and do not speak any of the four national languages. The family comprises a three-year-old daughter, an 11-year-old son, and the parents. There are three subsets of bilingualism which are classified as follows:

(a) **Compound**

The three-year-old has been learning the native language of the parents, and in Singapore, she attends a preschool and is immersed in English. She readily picks up the second language and begins to process the world around her in this language. Her command of English is excellent, and she might even pick up a local Singlish accent. However, as time passes, even children who are proficient in two languages begin to become more dominant in one language. It should not be seen as a problem because there are many benefits to bilingualism (see below). This early childhood form of bilingualism is known as "compound".

(b) **Coordinate**

The teenage brother speaks his native language, but in Singapore, he has to learn English from scratch. Fortunately, he picks it up very quickly. At school, he would speak English to his schoolmates, but at home, he might continue conversing in his native tongue. Over the years, he might speak English predominantly. His bilingualism is referred to as "coordinate".

(c) **Subordinate**

The parents are learning a secondary language but filters it through their primary native language. They sometimes have to think for a brief moment in order to understand what is said, translate the English heard or read into their native language and then translate it back to English, in order to express their thoughts. They may retain elements of an accent related to their native tongue. This form of bilingualism is known as "subordinate".

Because many bilingual individuals can become quite proficient in the new language, and barely colour the speech with their native accents or pronunciations, the difference in their speech may not even be apparent to a casual observer.

The brain[4]

How does the brain handle bilingualism? Functional magnetic resonance imaging and positron emission tomography scans have shown increased connectivity between the frontal and posterior parts of the brain compared with monolingual people, thus enhancing brain activity as well as cognitive reserve.

In early childhood, the brain is more malleable than an adult's and this plasticity allows the developing brain to use both right and left hemispheres in language acquisition. There is increased density of grey matter as well as more activity involving extensive areas of the brain including the frontal, parietal, and both left and right temporal lobes. Thus, learning of a second language by a very young child will activate many areas of the brain. In contrast, when learning a second language in adulthood, the brain development is largely confined to the left hemisphere only.

Creole or pidgin language[5,6]

In countries where more languages are spoken, there is a tendency for the speaker to combine two or more languages. This is referred to as creole or pidgin language. This has been divided into three classes according to the degree of "severity":

(a) Acrolect: This is considered "mild", where there is no significant difference between the spoken language from its origins, so listeners have no difficulty understanding the speaker.

(b) Mesolect: Also known as "moderate", this is the case where there are several loan words, plus some dropping of indefinite articles and plural markings on some nouns. Examples of mesolect include "sabo" = "sabotage", "shiok" = "great" (from the Malay language).

(c) Basilect: Considered the most "severe", where the combination of words from two or more languages is so "severe" that foreign listeners have difficulty understanding what is being spoken. This is referred to as heavy creole or heavy pidgin. An example is "I buay tahan he talk cock" which translates as "I cannot tolerate the nonsense he is talking."

Many speakers of heavy creole or heavy pidgin languages have the ability to switch from this severe form of slang to acrolect or even to the pure speech of the language of origin.

Bilingualism and dyslexia[7]

The question often asked is whether or not bilingualism or multilingualism contributes to, or exacerbates dyslexia. Studies have shown that identifying dyslexia in children who are starting to learn a new language, is extremely difficult. Challenges with reading or writing a second language may be the result of basic intelligence, motivation, and frequency of usage of the new language. The consensus of opinion is that problems associated with bilingualism are distinct from dyslexia, and they coexist separately.

Benefits of bilingualism[8,9]

There are many benefits of learning another language especially at a very young age. This is backed up by scientific studies, and the bonuses include:

- Enhancing mental development
- Promoting greater focus, flexibility, problem-solving skills, and creativity
- Ordering food more easily from hawker centres and food courts
- Watching movies without subtitles
- Enhancing memory and delaying memory loss[10-12]

- Maintaining contact with family, the older generation
- Retaining cultural heritage
- Having fewer racial biases, achieving better multiracial integration, and making more friends
- Doing more overseas business

Bilingualism is a national policy in Singapore schools, and is compulsory in government schools. However, it has come under some criticism. The problem is that not everyone is good at learning a second language, and some struggle and suffer painfully. Another problem is that those who are good at learning languages are not encouraged to learn a third language, such as Malay, Korean, Japanese, or an Indian or European language. Learning extra languages should be encouraged for capable individuals, because it can enhance future careers and business entrepreneurship.

Disadvantages of bilingualism[13]

Studies have shown there are certain drawbacks to learning two languages at a young age.

- Infants raised hearing and speaking two languages take longer to begin saying their first words. The explanation for this is that the infant needs to pay more attention and recognise more words with different phonemes from different languages.
- Young children tend to mix up the languages they are being exposed to. While they might learn the languages more readily, it seems harder for them to know whether to use the words from this language or that.
- Their vocabulary is usually more restricted. Although the total number of words they know is greater than that of a monolingual speaker, the number of words spoken in each separate language is fewer.

On balance, we can say that the benefits of bilingualism are greater than monolingualism, and that the disadvantages are only temporary. This sentiment is also echoed by language teachers and professional translators.

Will modern technology discourage learning another language?[14]

Currently, there are many devices that can automatically translate spoken words from one language to another. This means that there is no need to learn a foreign language. It is claimed that even culture-specific swear words, jargon, and slang are all translatable. So the question one will ask is: "Why bother learning another language?" The answer is that present-day devices may not be very good in translating the underlying emotions that accompany one's speech. The subtle subtext can be lost. For example, when one says something sarcastic like, "You think you are very clever?" it might be translated in a neutral way that the listener might even take as a compliment!

Conclusions

Bilingualism is an important ability that has many benefits, ranging from enhancing brain function to communicating with a wider range of people, delaying dementia, and enhancing overseas business. The younger a second language is introduced to a child, the better the long-term outcome. This is shown by the better command of the second language, and these individuals will be more flexible and creative in their thinking. Although bilingualism does not increase one's intelligence, it does delay Alzheimer Disease. It has been shown that even if you did not have the good fortune of learning a second language in early childhood, there are still benefits to learning one later in life. It exercises the brain, and as the saying goes, even "a little exercise can go a long way!" Finally, one last quote from Geoffrey Willans: "You can never understand one language until you understand at least two."

References

1. Costa A. The bilingual brain. Penguin Books 2017. ISBN 978-0-141-99038-5.
2. Wikipedia. Multilingualism. https://en.wikipedia.org/wiki/Multilingualism
3. Wikipedia. Neuroscience of multilingualism. https://en.wikipedia.org/wiki/Neuroscience_of_multilingualism

4. Goksan S *et al*. Early childhood bilingualism: effects on brain structure and function. F1000Research 2020. https://www.ncbi.nlm.nih.gov/pmc/articles/PMC7262573/

5. Nordquist R. Definition and examples of acrolects in language. ThoughtCo 2019. https://www.thoughtco.com/what-is-acrolect-1689057

6. Honeycombers. Singlish 101. The top Singlish phrases you must know to chat like a local. Honeycombers 2021. https://thehoneycombers.com/singapore/singlish-101/

7. McBride C. For children with dyslexia, multilingualism can be beneficial. Bold 2018. https://bold.expert/for-children-with-dyslexia-multilingualism-can-be-beneficial/

8. Skibba R. How a second language can boost the brain. Knowable Magazine 2018. https://knowablemagazine.org/article/mind/2018/how-second-language-can-boost-brain

9. Singh Leher. The benefits of bilingualism go beyond knowing two languages. CNA 2018. https://www.channelnewsasia.com/news/singapore/commentary-bilingualism-mother-tongue-language-benefits-9984098

10. Marian V & Shook A. The cognitive effects of being bilingual. Cerebrum 2012. https://dana.org/article/the-cognitive-benefits-of-being-bilingual/

11. Blom E *et al*. The benefits of being bilingual: Working memory in bilingual Turkish–Dutch children. Journal of Experimental Child Psychology 2014; 128: 105–119. https://www.sciencedirect.com/science/article/pii/S0022096514001180

12. Wodniecka Z *et al*. Does bilingualism help memory? Competing effects of verbal ability and executive control. International Journal of Bilingual Education and Bilingualism 2010; 13: 575–595. https://www.researchgate.net/publication/266617722_Does_bilingualism_help_memory_Competing_effects_of_verbal_ability_and_executive_control

13. Blarlo. Advantages and disadvantages of bilingualism. https://blog.blarlo.com/en/advantages-and-disadvantages-of-bilingualism/

14. Gadgets Reviews. Best voice translator devices on the market. Gadgets Reviews 2022. https://gadgets-reviews.com/review/1767-best-voice-translator-devices.html

10 Music

Introduction[1,2]

Music is a creative art form. We all have our own preferences as to the types of music we listen to. For example, we might choose the music of our childhood or culture, or we might go for classical, jazz, pop, hip hop or other styles of music.

Music is all around us. It is there when we turn on the radio or television, we might listen to it when studying or working, it is heard in shopping centres and food courts, it motivates our exercise work-outs, and we hear it on TikTok, YouTube and Spotify.

Music affects us emotionally, intellectually and bodily at many levels. It can convey sophisticated complex meanings, excite us with rhythms and harmonies, and it can soothe troubled spirits. It can unite us in intimate connections with others or allow us to sequester into the personal world of our imagination. Music has incredible powers to evoke memories of particular times, places, and people from our past. We dare say that of all the arts, music touches our soul most profoundly.

But how does music affect our minds?

What are the effects of music?[3]

Depending on the type of music listened to, researchers have discovered that the outcomes can be variable. However, if the music is specially chosen by the test subject, or if pleasant background music is played, the results are more often positive. Below are listed some of the effects that music may have on individuals:

1. **Increases Intelligence: The Mozart Effect[4,5]**

   In 1993, a provocative paper was published where 36 college students listened to a piece of Mozart and were then tested on their abstract reasoning and spatial abilities. Those who listened to Mozart performed better in a multiple choice test, a pattern analysis test and a paper folding and cutting test. However, the improvement only lasted less than 15 minutes. The researchers speculated that the enhanced performance was due to the complex music that stimulated the brain's spatial, analytical and abstract reasoning. Publication of this study saw parents worldwide hopping onto the bandwagon and playing Mozart to their children including unborn foetuses inside the womb, in the belief that music could enhance intelligence. Attempts to duplicate the results of this study have been inconsistent. More recent neurophysiological studies using neurochemical methods and function magnetic resonance imaging have shown that listening to music, including Mozart, raised the blood level of dopamine by 9 per cent, and increased activity in several areas of the brain that lasted up to 15 minutes. These studies show that music does have some physiological effects, which may possibly explain the Mozart Effect on some elements of the IQ test.

   More recently, there have been several studies attempting to see if music can have a direct effect on raising intelligence in children. For example, there was a study undertaken in a group of children aged four to six years who participated in a one-hour computer-based training programme with animated projections and colourful cartoons. Half were exposed to music while the other half only heard non-musical sounds. After four weeks, the children exposed to music tested higher on verbal IQ tests involving word recall, information analysis, and language-based reasoning. Other studies also showed that children who regularly listened to music or played musical instruments had a higher verbal and mathematical IQ compared to age-matched controls who were not exposed to music. It appears that listening to popular music is better at achieving this than hearing Mozart!

2. **Improves Memory[6,7]**

   Listening to music can trigger memories, sometimes with astonishing details. Exactly how this is accomplished is still speculative. Here are some possible reasons:
   - Reduces stress
   - Elevates your mood

- Clears up your thinking
- Increases alertness
- Gives you a rest period

3. **Improves Concentration and Attention**[8,9]

Instrumental music with a simple monotonous beat and a tune that an individual likes can improve one's focus. In contrast, loud songs, jazz, or grating heavy beat pop music can be off-putting and distracts one from studying or working. It is thought that background music might prevent environmental noises from becoming distracting, it may have a calming effect which enables the person to pay better attention, or perhaps, it clears the mind so that information is retained better.

4. **Increases Creativity**[10,11]

Researchers made subjects listen to different styles of music: one that made them happy, while other pieces of music made them sad, calm, and anxious respectively, and a final group of subjects merely sat in silence. The results showed the group that listened to happy music displayed more flexibility in their thinking and found more solutions to their tasks compared to the other groups.

5. **Helps Relieve Anxiety**[12,13]

Studies have shown that when people listen to the music they prefer, or to relaxing music, their level of psychological stress and anxiety are reduced significantly. One study used stressful situations that included normal childbirth and surgery. They found that subjects listening to music saw a greater rise in two stress-relieving hormones, namely cortisol and alpha-amylase. It is suggested that when an individual is facing high levels of stress, music might divert the focus away from the problem and thereby reduce anxiety.

6. **Music and Language**[14,15]

Language is largely processed in the left brain whereas music affects nearly all areas of the brain. Music has been shown to enhance language learning. It is thought that music sharpens one's discernment of pitch and helps in the appreciation of rhythms and the quality or timbre of sounds, which are important in both music and speech.

7. **Provides Coping Mechanisms**[16,17]

Studies have shown that music can change the perception of time passage. Fast tunes seem to speed up time, whereas slow tunes seem to slow it down.

8. **Helps Pain Control**[18,19]

Multiple studies have shown that when patients who have experienced injuries or recovering from surgery experience less pain when played their favourite songs. They also feel more comfortable, less anxious and tired, and more energetic. Music alleviates all levels of suffering, and appears to inspire healing.

9. **Learning a Musical Instrument Improves Motor Skills**[20]

Playing a musical instrument helps children develop fine motor skills. Dancing to music can also bring about higher levels of arm and leg motor control. These physical actions are stored in long-term memory.

10. **Strengthens Social Bonds**[21]

Music enhances socialising by bringing people together either to listen to music, sing in a choir or play in a band. It is a universal part of celebrations, parties, weddings, and concerts. Music increases one's empathy and enables one to see things from another person's point of view, also known as the "theory of mind". When people share the same appreciation of the same musical styles or genres, they show greater social cohesion. Music has also been demonstrated to increase the "love" or "feel good" hormone, which increases social connections.

11. **Helps Heart Disease**[22]

Music has been shown to reduce blood pressure, slow down heart rates and reduce anxiety. The combined effects of all these effects result in lowering the risk for heart attacks.

The neuroscience of music[23,24]

The eardrum can sense the pitch and melody of music, and the signals are transmitted first to the two auditory centres which are located in the temporal lobes on both sides of the brain. This first step is important because it evokes an emotional response.

The signal is then further transmitted to other areas of the brain. The lyrics of a song are processed in the left frontal cortex. The rhythm and timing of a piece of music is done in the frontal and parietal cortex, the cerebellum as well as the basal ganglia.

A signal is also sent to the nucleus accumbens which is located deep in the brain and is part of the basal ganglia. This nucleus releases dopamine, the chemical that makes a person feel good. This is the biochemical mechanism of the soothing effects of music.

Another signal is sent to the amygdala which is attached to the basal ganglia, and when activated, it sends a nervous impulse to the skin, so one can feel chills, goosebumps, or the hairs standing up on the back of the neck.

When a person starts singing, plays an instrument, or goes dancing, the motor cortex is activated.

Development of musical skills[25]

We have long known that for language development, there is a critical time at which a child learns to speak, read and write. The same goes for music. Unborn foetuses exposed to music can recognise the same music after birth. Caregivers might sing lullabies or play music to their babies. The styles of music may have some long-term influences in the behaviours and preferred music in later life. For example when played music from one's culture, one may appreciate it more. Depending on their age, children listen to a wide variety of music, ranging from children's lullabies to K-pop, rock, punk, hip hop, jazz, and classical music.

Children develop different aspects of music appreciation at different ages:

- Newborns respond to simple music beats
- 4-month-olds: Develop metrical structures common in their culture
- 6-month-olds: Recognise different melodies and melodic contours even when presented at a different pitch and tempo
- 9-month-olds: Spontaneous babbling or singing sounds
- 18-month-olds: Sing recognisable songs
- 2-year-olds: Spontaneous singing keeping to a rhythmic beat and start trying to move or dance to the musical pulse
- 3-year-olds: Sing songs but the melody may not be too accurate
- 4-year-olds: Melody increases in accuracy
- 5-year-olds: Can reproduce songs quite accurately and keep to a steady beat; Some may even start improvising or inventing songs
- Teenage years: Music may act as a badge of identity and those who prefer certain genres of music might form their own groups

Music therapy[26]

Music has a whole spectrum of positive effects as listed above, Therefore, it is expected that one can utilise music as a form of therapy. Over the years, it has been employed as a supplement to assist other treatments or therapies.

We can define music therapy as the discerning use of music to maintain, promote and restore emotional as well as physical health. It enhances the following:

- Auditory discrimination
- Fine motor skills
- Speech vocabulary
- Non-reasoning skills
- Memory

It is currently being used as adjunct therapy for a variety of disorders that include the following:

- Autism
- Depression
- Anxiety
- Schizophrenia
- Pain relief
- Pregnancy and delivery
- Parkinson Disease
- Stroke rehabilitation
- Slowing down dementia and Alzheimer Disease
- Cancer therapy

In the case of childhood autism, it appears that music improves social interactions, communication and social adaptation skills. Music also improves depressive symptoms as well as anxiety. In the case of surgery and intensive care, music therapy has a beneficial effect on anxiety, thereby reducing the need for medication. Pain relief is somewhat more controversial and the results are mixed.

How music therapy works is currently being explored using newer methods of evaluating brain functions. To date, music therapy is thought to take advantage of the brain's neuroplasticity by rewiring neural connections. In young children, it might also help by pruning some of "redundant" nerves. There is evidence that music therapy increases blood flow and increases dopamine in certain areas of the brain, resulting in helping not only music activity, but also enhancing speech understanding.

Music education

Throughout the world, many schools have withdrawn music and the arts from the formal school curriculum. Several reasons have been given. Some say that there are too few jobs open to musicians and artists. Others claim that cuts in school budgets leave no money for arts education. Students and parents may opt to stay clear of music and the arts because it is more difficult to score A's in these subjects compared to the sciences and mathematics. The net result is that children are deprived of the benefits of music, including enhancing creative thinking, better communication and socialising, relaxation and happiness. It is recommended that schools should reinstate music and the arts into the official educational syllabus.

Conclusions

When we hear music, we are often stimulated to produce more music, like singing, playing an instrument, drumming, or we may be fired up into swaying or dancing. Music can make us cheerful or melancholic, it can calm us down when we are agitated, and it can have emotional healing properties.

Indeed, music can change our lives. That is the power of music.

References

1. Hallam S. The psychology of music. Routledge 2019. ISBN-13: 978-1138098541.
2. Margulis EH. The psychology of music. Oxford University Press 2018. ISBN-13: 978-0190640156.

3. Schafer T *et al*. The psychological functions of music listening. Frontiers in Psychology 2013; 4: 511. https://www.ncbi.nlm.nih.gov/pmc/articles/PMC3741536/

4. Rauscher FH *et al*. Music and spatial task performance. Nature 1993; 365: 611.

5. Incadence. The Mozart effect. Incadence 2021. https://www.incadence.org/post/the-mozart-effect-explaining-a-musical-theory

6. Fabiny A. Music can boost memory and mood. Harvard Health Publishing 2015. https://www.health.harvard.edu/mind-and-mood/music-can-boost-memory-and-mood

7. Second Wind Movement. 9 Music and Memory Studies, Plus Key Take-aways. Second Wind Movement. https://secondwindmovement.com/music-and-memory/

8. Burnett D. Does music really help you concentrate? The Guardian 2016. https://www.theguardian.com/education/2016/aug/20/does-music-really-help-you-concentrate

9. Unify Health Team. Does music help you focus and concentrate more effectively? Unify Health Team 2019. https://unifyhealthlabs.com/music-help-focus-concentrate/

10. Vine B. Creative listening: how music can boost your creativity. Brain-World 2019. https://brainworldmagazine.com/creative-listening-music-can-boost-creativity/

11. Suttie J. How music helps us be more creative. Greater Good Science Center 2017. https://greatergood.berkeley.edu/article/item/how_music_helps_us_be_more_creative

12. Collins D. The power of music to reduce stress. PsychCentral 2021. https://psychcentral.com/stress/the-power-of-music-to-reduce-stress

13. Thoma MV *et al*. The effect of music on the human stress response. PLOS ONE. 2013; 8: e70156. https://pubmed.ncbi.nlm.nih.gov/23940541/

14. Liisi. How music helps language development. Weareteacherfinder 2019. https://blog.weareteacherfinder.com/blog/music-helps-language-development/

15. Paterson J. Can listening to music help your child with language develop-ment and reading comprehension? PsychCentral 2016. https://psychcentral.com/lib/can-listening-to-music-help-your-child-with-language-development-and-reading-comprehension#1

16. Garrido S. Music and trauma: the relationship between music, trauma, per-sonality and coping style. Frontiers in Psychology 2015; 6: 977. https://www.frontiersin.org/articles/10.3389/fpsyg.2015.00977/full

17. Phillips CS & Woods HL. A musical approach to coping with psychosocial stress. American Nurse 2021. https://www.myamericannurse.com/a-musical-approach-to-coping-with-psychosocial-stress/

18. Klassen JA et al. Music for pain and anxiety in children undergoing medical procedures. Ambulatory Pediatrics 2008; 8: 117–128. https://www.sciencedirect.com/science/article/abs/pii/S1530156707002857?via%3Dihub

19. Holden R & Holden J. Music: a better alternative than pain? British Journal of General Practice 2013; 63: 536. https://www.ncbi.nlm.nih.gov/pmc/articles/PMC3782778/

20. Forgeard M et al. Practicing a Musical Instrument in Childhood is Associated with Enhanced Verbal Ability and Nonverbal Reasoning. PLOS ONE 2008. https://journals.plos.org/plosone/article?id=10.1371/journal.pone.0003566

21. Suttie J. Four ways music strengthens social bonds. Greater Good Magazine 2015. https://greatergood.berkeley.edu/article/item/four_ways_music_strengthens_social_bonds

22. Harvard Health Publishing. Using music to tune the heart. Harvard Health Publishing 2019. https://www.health.harvard.edu/newsletter_article/using-music-to-tune-the-heart

23. Wikipedia. The neuroscience of music. https://en.wikipedia.org/wiki/Neuroscience_of_music

24. Ginsborg J. The psychological results of music on the mind. HapidzFadli 2022. https://www.insure4music.co.uk/blog/2021/06/02/the-psychological-effects-of-music-on-the-brain/

25. Dumont E et al. Music interventions and child development. Frontiers in Psychology 2017; 8: 1694. https://www.ncbi.nlm.nih.gov/pmc/articles/PMC5626863/

26. Novotney A. Music as medicine. Monitor on Psychology 2013. https://www.apa.org/monitor/2013/11/music

11 Personality

Introduction

A parent commented: "How come my children are so different even though they have the same parents and have been brought up in the same household? One is so quiet and carefree, while another runs around continuously, and a third is bubbly and sociable. Their personalities are so dissimilar. Why?"

Every one of us has a different, unique persona. Even children have their own different characters, and they have difficulty hiding their personality. The environment also plays a role. When in a new place, a child may be a bit withdrawn, but once they become accustomed to the place, they will display their natural temperament.

What makes us different is our brains. Our brains control our senses, our acquisition of knowledge and experiences, our interpretation of the world, our emotions, and our expressions of thoughts and movements.

What is personality?[1]

Personality is the sum total of the attributes or qualities that form an individual's distinctive character. It is made up of a set of behaviours, understandings, and emotional patterns that affect one's motivations and the psychological interactions with others.

Our personality is not constant. It is shaped throughout our lives, especially during our childhood and youth, and it alters when our environment changes. For example, parents have often observed that their child's behaviour transforms from a rowdy extrovert at home into a quiet introvert at school.

What are the elements that comprise personality?[2]

To dissect the individual components that form the fundamental basis of personality, there are a number of different approaches, but only three major approaches will be discussed here, namely the:

(a) The Four Humours of Hippocrates,
(b) The Neuropsychological Approach,
(c) The Traits Theory (which includes the Big Five Personality Traits).

(a) The Four Humours of Hippocrates

Historically, the oldest proposition is by Hippocrates (460–377 BC), who suggested that human personality is made up of four humours or temperaments:

- Sanguine: optimistic courageous, sociable, energetic, disorganised
- Phlegmatic: unemotional, slow, meek, submissive, trustworthy
- Choleric: bad-tempered, explosive, dominant, confident, overbearing
- Melancholic: sad, depressed, moody, sensitive, thoughtful

Frank Baum's Wizard of Oz

Some people have tried to fit Frank Baum's (1856–1919) characters from The Wizard of Oz into these four humours. The lion is placed in the sanguine category, but initially he is a coward and he only discovers his courage towards the end. The tin man is unemotional and therefore phlegmatic. Dorothy is upset because she had lost her way home, and at a stretch, can be said to be choleric. The scarecrow is melancholic and sad, and he thinks he is worthless.

(b) The Neuropsychological Approach[3]

It is recognised that all our thinking, behaviours and responses are governed by our brains. Thus, one method of analysing personality is using a neuropsychological scientific analysis of brain functions. Using electroencephalography, functional magnetic resonance imaging, positron emission tomography, and pharmaco-biochemical responses, we can discover the parameters that determine personality.

(c) **The Traits Theory[4]**

This is one of the major approaches exploring the components or traits that make up personality. This is subdivided into:

- Cardinal traits: These are traits that dominate one's entire personality. They include integrity, generosity, narcissism, kindness, ambition and self-control. Cardinal traits can be both positive or negative and become more evident in older children.
- Central traits: These are the general characteristics that form the basic foundation of personality. They include intelligence and dullness, outspokenness and shyness, honesty and deceit, being carefree and anxious.
- Secondary traits: These are related to attitudes or preferences. They are usually expressed only in specific situations or certain circumstances. Stage fright, or impatience while waiting in line are examples of secondary traits.

The Big Five Personality Traits (modified for children)[5,6]

A popular subtype of the Traits Theory is the so-called Big Five, or a set of personality-building features:

1. **Conscientiousness (Persistent)**

   These are children who keep asking questions incessantly: "Why", "how", "how come". They are hungry for knowledge and will tell you in detail what they have been doing at school. Highly inquisitive, they also love to share the information they have gleaned and can be very creative. They are good at planning, and can keep to a timetable. Many of these children do well in their studies, and grow up to become original thinkers, inventors, writers, scientists and engineers.

   The opposite trait is the child who is lazy, undisciplined, and careless.

2. **Extraversion (Socializer)**

   Children with this trait are very sociable and talkative. They make friends easily and like to play with other children of all ages. They are fun-loving, cheerful, and like to dress up, pretend play and grab attention. Sometimes, they can be a bit aggressive. Many grow up to become actors, dancers, singers, and entrepreneurs.

The opposite are introverts, who are more quiet, serious, and withdrawn. Famous introverts include Albert Einstein and Isaac Newton.

3. **Agreeableness (Kind-hearted)**
These children are kind and sensitive. They are willing to share their toys and if they see a friend or an animal looking sad, they will try to comfort them. They are cooperative, empathetic, warm, and trusting. These children can grow up to become health care or social workers, musicians, artists and mathematicians.

The opposite are those who are competitive, ruthless, irritable and vindictive.

4. **Openness (Adventurous)**
You will encounter children who will explore parks and playgrounds, ride a bike as well as and try new foods and activities. They do not need much encouragement to engage in something daring and inventive. Many of them will have bumps and bruises all over and look like a wild child. Some might grow up to become leaders, entrepreneurs, and innovators.

The opposite are the conventional, pragmatic, realistic, conventional child who is unwilling to try anything new.

5. **Neuroticism (Worrier)**
These are children who worry a lot. They are anxious about everything, are uncertain if they should try something new. They cry easily and become depressed.

The opposite are children who are more resilient, even-keeled, relaxed, and have high self-esteem.

Preferred approach to personality

Which is the best way to look at personality? There are no correct answers to this question. The problem is that human personalities are so diverse and complex that there is no one best way of analysing this subject matter.

Each approach has its own merits. The neuropsychological perspective is very scientific and opens a lot of information doors about brain functions, but it is too cold and distant and does not provide the insight that we seek when trying to assess the personality of a person.

Personality tests[7,8]

There have been several tests that attempt to analyse and categorise one's personality type. Some companies use them to determine whom to employ. Some mental health professionals might use the tests to aid in the diagnosis and management of psychopathological personality disorders. Most members of the public probably take these tests out of curiosity to see if the tests can accurately capture their personality.

We will just look at three popular personality tests:

    (a) The Minnesota Multiphasic Personality Inventory (MMPI),

    (b) the Myers-Briggs Type Indicator (MBTI), and

    (c) The Enneagram.

(a) **Minnesota Multiphasic Personality Inventory (MMPI)[9]**

Introduced in 1948 at the University of Minnesota, it has since undergone several revisions. It is the most scientifically evaluated and comprehensive personality test. In addition, it evaluates psychopathology. This test is given to subject above the age of 14 years.

(b) **Myers-Briggs Type Indicator (MBTI)[10]**

Inspired by Carl Jung's (1875–1961) Psychological Types, this test was constructed by Katherine Briggs and her daughter Isabel Myers, and they published their Type Indicator Handbook in 1944. The test has been modified over the years and renamed the Myers-Briggs Type Indicator. It was originally recommended that the test be administered to subject above the age of 14 years. The foundation of the MBTI is the tenet that there are four dimensions or dichotomies of how people perceive the world and make decisions. Each dichotomy creates a scale. The four dichotomies are:

1. Introvert vs. Extrovert

2. Sensing vs. Intuitive

3. Thinking vs. Feeling
4. Perceiving vs. Judging

The permutations and combinations of these four dimensions yield 16 personality types. Interestingly, the four scales used in the MBTI have some correlation with four of the Big Five personality traits, which are currently more accepted than the MBTI.

(c) **The Enneagram**[11]

The Enneagram system of personality types has come under a barrage of criticism, including the lack of rigorous scientific validation and its links to mysticism. Using a nine-pointed star chart, it divides people into nine types, and everyone belongs to one type all of one's life.

Criticisms of personality tests[12]

One important attack on the validity of personality tests was made by the psychologist Walter Mischel. After reviewing dozens of studies on personality tests, he discovered that the results of many personality tests, including the MBTI and Enneagram, are not consistent. Up to 47 per cent of testers end up with a different personality type when retested. He argued that if there is reasonable stability in personality traits, then the wild fluctuations in typing must be due to a flawed test.

Defenders of personality tests

Defenders of personality tests would point to all biological tests, such as blood pressure or tests of attention deficit hyperactivity, as having some degree of inconsistency. There will be fluctuations in the results depending on the time of day, or day of the week the test is conducted. It is argued that for a test like the MBTI, if the test subject is someone who is emotional or aggressive, then they are naturally more prone to variations in their tests; it may also depend on environmental circumstances. The test itself, it is maintained, is good, and there is nothing wrong with it. Furthermore, it is sensitive enough to reflect a person's constant changes in personality. After all, people behave differently at school, in the office, in a party, in a religious environment, with family members, and so on. The problem is that individuals get bored with repeated tests, and they can become capricious with multiple testing, and perhaps, some may even sabotage them. Conscious and unconscious factors which can affect the expression of different aspects of personality, especially during testing, are not taken into account with these studies.

Other attacks on personality tests

A common attack levelled against personality testing is that personality is like a huge metaphorical elephant. We do not fully understand the nature of the beast. And the current state of the art in testing is still in its infancy. Thus, each test conducted is rather like a blind person feeling a different part of this proboscidean. People are too readily labelled as "individualist" or "challenger" or ESFJ (extroversion, sensing, feeling, judgment) or INTP (introversion, intuition, thinking, perceiving), or something else. Another attack is that the test subject can manipulate their answers thereby distorting their personality at will.

Personality labelling

It is true that personality labels are somewhat obscure and not well-defined. Are we justified in labelling people and then using the labels to predict their future behaviour, their future partnership or job suitability? Until we gain a much better understanding of personality, it would be too presumptuous to use these tests to determine someone's entire livelihood in the future. However, maybe one should not throw out the personality test baby with the entire testing bath water. One should continue to refine the tests.

Do we have multiple personalities?[13,14]

We all hate being typecast because we do not consider ourselves to be one-dimensional. It is possible that we all have multiple personalities. We mould our personality to match the person we are interacting with at that moment in time. As for career advice, we certainly do not wish to be told which profession is best for our personality (e.g. a garbage collector!).

However, there is an uncommon disorder of multiple personalities or dissociative personality disorder. Individuals with this condition have two or more distinct personality states that are usually long-lasting. Childhood traumatic events or child abuse may be the cause in some cases. Psychotherapy or cognitive behavioural therapy may help sometimes, but the condition usually persists.

Can you change your personality?[15,16]

The most famous change in personality is that of railroad worker Phineas Gage whose left frontal brain lobe was pierced by a metal rod in 1848. Before the accident, his fellow workers described him as "efficient and capable", but after the injury, he was said to be "fitful, irreverent, indulging at times in the grossest profanity (which was not previously his custom), manifesting but little deference for his fellows". He had become a moody, aggressive alcoholic and he could not stick with any job.

Another line of evidence that personality can change is a 2011 study, where people were given the hallucinogenic "magic mushroom", psilocybin. Subjects given this medicine therapeutically became more open, and could better withstand stresses.

It has also been observed that extroverted toddlers evolve into introverted adolescents. As individuals age further, they are gradually become more extroverted, less neurotic, more congenial and more meticulous. Personality changes have also been noted in Alzheimer Disease patients; in addition to memory loss, they also display apathy, agitation, aggression, delusions and depression. These changes have been reported by relatives and close friends.

Parenting styles[17]

Sometimes, there is a mismatch between a child's personality and that of the parents. The child may be more playful while the parent may be strict and obsessive. Conversely, the child may want to be alone, while the parent may want to socialise. This mismatch can lead to clashes.

Understand both your own as well as your child's temperament, and take a step back to look at the broader picture. Instead of becoming bothered and exasperated, try to think of some ways of solving the problem, or come up with compromises.

Keep your needs separate

Another common parenting challenge is that of separating parental needs and temperamental style from that of their children. A parent may believe that a child "needs" lots of social activity, for example, when in fact, the parent desires it. Being clear on your own parenting style and needs can help you maintain healthy boundaries and see your children as individuals.

Final notes

What makes us distinctive and individual is our personality. We know that the brain plays a major role in shaping our personality, but the precise way this is achieved remains a mystery. It is made up of a constellation of different traits which are assembled in an infinity of combinations and permutations to create a universe in our mind.

Each one of us is special.

References

1. Corr PJ & Matthews G. The Cambridge Handbook of Personality Psychology 2nd edition 2020. ISBN: 978-1108404457.
2. Wikipedia. Personality. https://en.wikipedia.org/wiki/Personality
3. Schretien DJ et al. A neuropsychological study of personality. Journal of Clinical and Experimental Neuropsychology 2010; 32: 1068–1973. https://www.ncbi.nlm.nih.gov/pmc/articles/PMC2937090/
4. Cherry K. What is the traits theory of personality? VeryWell Mind 2022. https://www.verywellmind.com/trait-theory-of-personality-2795955
5. Wikipedia. Big five personality traits. https://en.wikipedia.org/wiki/Big_Five_personality_traits
6. Cherry K. The big five personality traits. VeryWell Mind 2021. https://www.verywellmind.com/the-big-five-personality-dimensions-2795422
7. Wikipedia. Personality Tests. https://en.wikipedia.org/wiki/Personality_test
8. Harper H. The 23 best personality tests in ranking order. WorkStyle 2022. https://www.workstyle.io/best-personality-test

9. Framingham J. Minnesota Multiphasic Personality Inventory (MMPI). PsychCentral 2016. https://psychcentral.com/lib/minnesota-multiphasic-personality-inventory-mmpi#Development-of-the-MMPI

10. Moffa M. A critique of the Myers Briggs Type Indicator. Recruiter.com. https://www.recruiter.com/i/critique-of-the-myers-briggs-type-indicator-critique/ https://www.recruiter.com/recruiting/a-critique-of-the-myers-briggs-type-indicator-mbti-part-two/

11. Sloat S. Why one popular personality test is "pseudoscientific at best". Inverse 2020. https://www.inverse.com/mind-body/enneagram-personality-test-experts-explain

12. Voridis C. The Validity of Personality Tests: Criticism and Evaluation. LinkedIn 2016. https://www.linkedin.com/pulse/validity-personality-tests-criticism-evaluation-voridis/

13. Cherry, K. Phineas Gage: His Accident and Impact on Psychology. VeryWell Mind 2022. What is multiple personality disorder? https://www.verywellmind.com/phineas-gage-2795244

14. Wikipedia. Dissociative identity disorder. https://en.wikipedia.org/wiki/Dissociative_identity_disorder

15. Legg TJ. Everything you want to know about personality change. Healthline 2019. https://www.healthline.com/health/behavior-unusual-or-strange#causes

16. Gui-Evans O. Phineas Gage. Simply Psychology 2020. https://www.simplypsychology.org/phineas-gage.html

17. YouAreMom. Parenting styles and children's personalities. YouAreMom 2019. https://youaremom.com/children/parenting-styles/

12 Mental Health

Introduction[1-4]

The past few years have seen a significant rise in the number of children seeking psychological help for mental problems. Unfortunately, the COVID-19 pandemic has exacerbated this issue. The question being asked is whether we are tackling the challenge effectively. If not, why not? First, let us define what we mean by mental health in children.

Definition[5]

Mental health is the complete well-being of a person, including their emotional, psychological, and social life. This affects how one thinks, feels, and acts. It can determine how one handles stress, interacts with others, and makes choices.

A child's mental health is defined slightly differently from an adult's; it is more nuanced and multifaceted, and because of its inconsistent fragmentary manifestation, it is often overlooked or misdiagnosed as a normal variation. In addition to emotional and social aspects of psychological health, there are influences by behavioural and cognitive functions.

Each child travels along their own unique developmental path, and different experiences can affect their mental states and thinking over time. A young child may not understand what they have done wrong and why you are reprimanding them. Also, they may not be able to express themselves to tell you what they are feeling. Children's mental health is a continuum, stretching from early childhood all the way to adulthood, so the definition of mental health needs to embrace the different emotions and expressions associated with the different stages of life.

Presentation[6,7]

It is often said that young children wear their hearts on their sleeves. Certainly, children may not be able to hide their feelings very well. When upset, they will cry. In contrast, a late teenager's thinking resembles more of an adult's than a child's in that they can hide their feelings. It is therefore a challenge for parents, teachers and doctors to learn how to decipher a child's behaviour and figure out their underlying meaning.

Changes in behaviour are still the best clues in assessing mental disorders. If a very outgoing sociable young child suddenly becomes reclusive, refuses to eat, does not want to go to school, or refuses to do what they normally do, then something may be wrong. If they are normally close to their parents and undergo a massive change in behaviour by becoming inconsistent, or shun spending time to talk to or hug their loved ones, then it is time to delve a little deeper.

Mental health problems of older children and teenagers may be more difficult to detect because they may look perfectly healthy at first glance, until you look more closely at their facial expressions or body language. There are certain societal norms that, when crossed, may provide clues to potential behavioural abnormalities. For example, if a child becomes inappropriately happy, sad or angry given the circumstances, this can be a clue. Here is a list of the more common signs and symptoms suggestive of mental health problems:

- Lying awake all night
- Eating too much
- Feeling sad or depressed
- Lack of interest or motivation
- Feeling nervous or anxious
- Failing at school when previously doing well
- Withdrawal from social activities and sports
- Poor concentration, memory loss, illogical thinking
- Heightened sensitivity to sounds, sights, touch, smells
- Unusually odd, uncharacteristic behaviour

Prevalence[8]

The prevalence of mental health problems in Singapore has been found to be 13.9 per cent which is lower than the global average of 20 per cent, but is nevertheless quite a burden. However, the prevalence has increased during the COVID-19 pandemic.

Psychiatrists have reported an increased number of referrals for mental health issues during the COVID-19 pandemic.[9]

Causes

Failing at school tests or exams, scolded by teachers, being bullied at school or cyberbullied on the internet, emotional abuse by friends, can all precipitate mental problems. On top of that, there may be parental conflicts, or other family problems resulting from job losses and reduced financial income. Additional factors include suspension of overseas vacations, limitations of entertainment in cinema and theatre because of a reduction in seating capacity, and the inability to dine out with larger numbers, which have added further to mental stress.

Neurodevelopmental causes

What causes mental health impairments? Twenty-first century science is exploring the answers at a molecular level, where genetics play a crucial role. Brain function results from an interaction between genes and environmental experiences. This interchange affects mental health, behaviour, personality, and other neurological functions. Exactly how genes and environment interact to regulate our neurodevelopmental operating systems remains a mystery.

Physical diseases such as infections and injuries, as well as side effects of drugs, alcohol and substance abuse, can affect the developing brain and lead to long-term behavioural and emotional problems. What is less certain is how emotional stress, inappropriate parenting, and poor school teaching, can destabilise neuronal connections and lead to mental health problems. The influence of peers may play a key role in mental health as well. We are also aware that watching movies, television, playing computer games and spending too much time on the Internet can all play a part in affecting our emotions.

Management

One cannot tell if a child has mental health problems merely by looking at them. To the outside world, they may look perfectly normal. Feeling sad, angry, or stressed are all a part of life, just as it is normal to feel happy, confident and carefree sometimes. Positive and negative emotions come and go, depending on what is happening around that person. How do we tell if a child is having significant emotional problems? And if they do have such problems, how do we restore them back to good mental health? Here are some steps that practitioners have recommended for both the child as well as the adult:

- **Talk**
  This is the most important step to take. Talk to your child and listen to their feelings and thoughts without any pressure or judgement. Sometimes, overwhelming feelings are brought on by events in one's life; sometimes, they happen for no reason at all, and it may be helpful to talk about these emotions. For the older child, who hears imaginary voices, rather than becoming frightened, it is sometimes helpful to accept and communicate with these voices, sharing thoughts and ideas. It may sound unorthodox, but some have found this tactic useful. Alternatively, you can communicate with them via social media. Choose whom you talk to carefully.
- **Exercise**
  One of the best tools for treating anxiety and mild depression is physical exercise. Help your child exercise at home, or play indoor or outdoor sports. If the gym is open, you can go there regularly. Even if you are in a lockdown or on stay-home notice, you can try to get some fresh air on the balcony. But if it is possible, go outdoors for exercise and walks.
- **Take a Break**
  Take a break and do something your child enjoys: drink a hot drink, watch Netflix, play with a pet, or whatever makes you and your child feel better.

- **Express Your Feelings and Thoughts**
  Encourage your child to write a journal or a blog, write some poetry, do some art, music, or photography, start a vlog, or post a dance on TikTok.
- **Volunteer to Help Others**
  Volunteer for social services. You and your child can help deliver food and groceries to disadvantaged people, give online tuition for the underprivileged, or learn to be a mental health advocate.
- **Mindfulness**
  You can practise mindfulness or do some yoga and meditate. Some people are helped by this.
- **Consult a Professional**
  If you or your child are still feeling down, you might consider consulting someone else who might be able to give some professional advice. It can be a family member, a teacher, a health professional, or a spiritual advisor.
- **Limit Access to the daily News**
  "No news is good news." Currently, most of the news on television and newspapers tend to focus on bad news, such as the spread of COVID-19 and the mortality rate. Therefore, it may be advisable to restrict one's access and time to listen to the news.

Educating parents, caregivers and teachers

The issue of educating caregivers lies at the root of adult emotional literacy. Our education system has not educated future parents to be good parents. They are not taught the optimal response to their child's misbehaviour, temper tantrums, and refusals. Asian parents are often viewed as being too strict with their children and may often resort to caning or physical punishment. Parents have not been schooled on various techniques like displaying empathy and compassion to a misbehaving child. Many parents discipline their children in the same way that they themselves had been disciplined during their own childhood.

How should parents respond to emotional problems or traumatic events? Should they reprimand a crying child and tell them to stop crying, or give them an angry look? Well, this might deter the child from expressing their feelings to the parents, and they will likely repress their emotions.

When this scolding recurs over time, the child might react in the form of aggression, rage, or shouting. Later, this can evolve into bullying behaviour, or even show up as violence. But if the child is doing something potentially dangerous, then it may be appropriate to shake one's head and give a stern look, and explain the danger of the situation.

When parents respond to their sad or crying child by saying: "It's OK for you to express how you feel. I will accept you as you are, the angry you, the sad you, as well as the happy you. Let me hold you for a moment." When you display empathy and compassion to your child, and show that the home is a safe place to be, then after they have calmed down, you can explain why you think they should behave in a more rational reasonable way.

However, if the child is crying because you have denied them something they want, then it is important not to capitulate and give in to them. This would encourage crying as a means to manipulate you to acquiesce to their future demands. Take time to explain why you cannot give your child what they want. Maybe you can give an alternative suggestion.

Educating parents, caregivers, and teachers is therefore an important part of child-rearing.

What about the education system?[10,11]

The other problem in many Asian countries is that parents value IQ more than EQ, and some even rate exam scores more highly than integrity. Over the years, the education system has become more rigid, more stressful, more hyper-competitive, and less enjoyable. It is becoming more like an Olympic Games sport that only gives you one chance to prove yourself. It is unforgiving. If you are knocked out in an early round, there is no second chance to allow for a comeback. Many parents send their children for extra tuition in order to gain an advantage in school exams.

No wonder most school children are frustrated and stressed. It makes them perpetually anxious and fatigued, and there is little enjoyment in school life. This can lead to further anxiety, sadness, and depression.

Children develop at different rates and some may be better at certain subjects and not others, and some might excel in non-academic subjects like the arts or sports. The rather unimaginative exam system, often using multiple choice questions, also limits creative thinking and adds more pressure on schoolchildren.

The stress of exams is a perennial problem. Children worry that they are falling behind in their revision. If they did well in a previous exam, then expectations are for them to do as well, if not better, in the next exam. And when they do badly, it is the similar feeling of having won an Olympic medal the last time but failing this time to defend your title. On top of your own disappointment is the added disappointment of your parents who harp on why you did not study harder and why you wasted your time on the Internet. Even if the parents kept quiet, the child automatically assumes that they are upset by poor exam results. These pressures can be overwhelming.

During the COVID-19 pandemic, children have had to spend less time at school and more time at home. Group activities like choirs, orchestras, team sports, theatre and celebrations have been curtailed. The inability for children to physically attend school during periods of pandemic lockdown, the restrictions preventing going outdoors and being stuck at home, the change in classroom teaching to home-based web learning, has had some adverse emotional impact because of the social isolation.

Suicide rates among school children saw a spike during this pandemic.[12] This requires urgent attention. Fortunately, Singapore and other countries are addressing this problem.[13-16]

Conclusions

Mental health of children, when managed in a sensitive, exemplary way, can lead to a well-balanced, selfless, ethical, humane person, someone capable of thinking critically and creatively. This requires careful appropriate care of children by parents, caregivers, teachers and friends. We recognise that each child is different, and that education needs to be individualised and customised for the different stages of child development. Much more attention must be devoted to this area of child development. Hopefully, changes will come soon.

Finally, there is a saying that mental health is an integral part of health, and that there is no health without mental health!

For information about mental health in Singapore, go to the Institute of Mental Health Singapore's website.[17] Also see Chapter 17 on Depression and Suicide.

References

1. Lebrun-Harris LA *et al.* Five-year trends in US children's health and well-being, 2016-2020. JAMA Pediatrics 2022. https://jamanetwork.com/journals/jamapediatrics/fullarticle/2789946

2. Jeffreys B. Children's mental health: huge rise in severe cases, BBC analysis reveals. BBC News 2022. https://www.bbc.com/news/education-60197150

3. Goh CT. The challenges young people face in seeking mental health help. CNA 2020. https://www.channelnewsasia.com/singapore/in-focus-young-people-mental-health-singapore-treatment-613566

4. Goh T. IMH study points to likely increase in mental health issues in S'pore amid Covid-19. The Straits Times 2021. https://www.straitstimes.com/singapore/health/imh-study-points-to-likely-increase-in-mental-health-issues-in-spore-amid-covid-19

5. Wikipedia. Mental health. https://en.wikipedia.org/wiki/Mental_health

6. Parekh, R. Warning signs of mental illness. American Psychiatric Association. https://www.psychiatry.org/patients-families/warning-signs-of-mental-illness

7. U.S. Department of Health & Human Services. What is mental health? U.S. Department of Health & Human Services 2022. https://www.mentalhealth.gov/basics/what-is-mental-health

8. Evlanova A. What is the state of mental health in Singapore? Yahoo Finance 2019. https://www.valuechampion.sg/what-state-mental-health-singapore

9. Ong A. Worries over COVID-19 situation are taking a mental toll on Singapore. CNA 2021. https://www.channelnewsasia.com/news/commentary/covid-19-coronavirus-singapore-mental-health-hotline-resource-14899148

10. Bouchrika I. 50 Current Student Stress Statistics: 2021/2022 Data, Analysis & Predictions. Research.com 2020. https://research.com/education/student-stress-statistics

11. Poh B. A hyper-competitive culture is breeding severe test anxiety among many students. CNA 2018. https://www.channelnewsasia.com/news/commentary/hyper-competitive-culture-breeding-severe-test-anxiety-among-10744150

12. Tham D. Suicide cases in Singapore highest in 8 years amid COVID-19 pandemic. CNA 2021. https://www.channelnewsasia.com/singapore/suicide-highest-record-elderly-mental-health-isolation-covid-19-1984716

13. Calland C & Hutchinson N. Tackling anxiety in schools. Routledge 2022. ISBN 9780367620974. https://www.routledge.com/Tackling-Anxiety-in-Schools-Lessons-for-Children-Aged-3-13/Calland-Hutchinson/p/book/9780367620974

14. Mellor A. How we can tackle the child mental health crisis. Tes Magazine 2022. https://www.tes.com/magazine/analysis/general/new-ways-thinking-about-schools-wellbeing-pupil-mental-health-has-real-impact

15. Lin C. MOE to strengthen support networks in schools; all teachers to get enhanced training on mental health literacy. CNA 2021. https://www.channelnewsasia.com/singapore/mental-health-schools-support-network-teachers-enhanced-training-2077836

16. Baker JA. Social service agencies to get more support to help youth with mental health issues. CNA 2022. https://www.channelnewsasia.com/singapore/youth-mental-health-issues-imh-social-service-agencies-training-support-2564951

17. Child Guidance Clinic Singapore. Institute of Mental Health. https://www.imh.com.sg/Clinical-Services/Outpatient-Clinics/Pages/Child-Guidance-Clinic.aspx

Other information

Getting help

National Care Hotline: 1800-202-6868 (8:00am to 12 noon)

Mental well-being

Mental Health Helpline: 6389-2222 (24 hours)
Samaritans of Singapore: 1800-221-4444 (24 hours)
Singapore Association for Mental Health: 1800-283-7019 (Mon to Fri, 9:00am to 6:00pm)
Silver Ribbon Singapore: 6386-1928, 6509-0271 (Mon to Fri, 9:00am to 6:00pm)
Tinkle Friend: 1800-274-4788 (Mon to Fri, 2:30 to 5:00pm)

Counselling

Touchline 1800-377-2252 (Mon to Fri, 9:00am to 6:00pm)
Care Corner Counselling Centre (Mandarin): 1800-353-5800 (10:00am to 10:00pm)

13 Intellectual disability

Introduction

Children follow a similar timetable for development, a given calendar for achieving motor, communication and social skills. Like the steps of a staircase, one climbs one step at a time.

Most children learn to walk and talk soon after their first birthday. They join two to four words into a phrase by two years, copy a circle by three years, and count up to 10 around four years old. Parents get very worried when their child does not reach these milestones at the expected time, and they might ask around to check if their child is developmentally delayed. They get even more worried when they hear that their child is suspected to be "intellectual disabled". What does this term mean?

Sidenote

Nobody likes to be stigmatised. Over the years, the words used to label people with developmental delay have changed several times. We try our best not to use language that might be perceived as being disparaging to these individuals. The terms "intellectual disability" or "intellectually challenged" are used in a neutral manner and are not meant to have any other connotations.

Definition[1-3]

Intellectual disability is an impairment of mental abilities that impacts adaptive functioning, with an onset during a person's developmental period (<22 years).

The definition of intellectual disability is based on two major assessments.

1. The IQ test
    The intellectual function is significantly below average when formally tested, with an IQ score of less than around 70. A lower IQ results in problems with one's abilities in learning, reasoning, and problem-solving.
2. Adaptive functioning
    Adaptive functioning concerns activities of daily life, communication and the ability to live independently. This is subdivided into conceptual, social and practical skills:
    *   Conceptual: Learning a language and literacy skills
        Ability to handle the concepts of numbers, money, and time
        Capability of self-direction so as to live independently
    *   Social   Interpersonal skills — the ability to make and keep friends
        Social responsibility
        Self-esteem
        Gullibility, naiveté
        Social problem-solving
    *   Practical Skills   Daily living activities, personal care
        Occupational skills, job responsibilities
        Healthcare
        Travel and transportation
        Able to manage recreation activities
        Use of money and the handphone

It should be pointed out that some of the features mentioned above are multifactorial and not easily classified into fixed categories.

IQ tests

The IQ score remains a major way of identifying persons who are intellectually challenged or disabled. There are several IQ tests available for children over the age of 1 year.[4] However, it is sometimes difficult to decide which test is the best. For children between the ages of 1 and 42 months, the Bayley Scales for Infant and Toddler Development is available; it measures development level, not IQ. For children above the age of six years, the Wechsler Intelligence Test for children (WISC) is popular. There is a modified WISC for children over the age of two years. The oldest test, the Stanford-Binet IQ test is also available and some psychologists are still using it.

The problem with conducting IQ tests on children is that their cooperation is essential, and if it is not forthcoming, the test is inaccurate. There is a discrepancy of five points either way using the same test on separate occasions. About 14 per cent of children's IQ will change by 10 points or more on follow up over a two-year period. Different IQ tests have shown scores that can vary by up to 12 points. Hence, the inaccuracy and instability of IQ test scores, especially when applied to children, makes one wonder about their reliability, and whether a wrong reading can be problematic.[5] Should we reconsider the use of IQ tests in the diagnosis of intellectual disability?[6]

Exclusionary criteria

Factors that can distort IQ testing include hearing or visual impairment, having attention deficit hyperactivity disorder (ADHD), dyslexia, or feeling sleepy. Therefore, to come to a more accurate diagnosis of intellectual disability, one must rule out the following:

- Visual, hearing or motor disability
- Autism, ADHD, dyslexia
- Emotional disturbances
- Cultural factors
- Environmental or economic disadvantages
- Limited proficiency in the language used for the IQ test

The IQ test should be conducted by an experienced qualified psychologist who can give appropriate instructions understood by the test subject. If the results are unclear, it may be necessary to repeat the assessment.

Levels of intellectual disability

It is traditional to classify the degree of intellectual impairment based on the IQ score, and one then tries to correlate the score with the degree of support the individual might requires in daily life:

- IQ 55–69 Mild   Intermittent support. Children with this level of IQ can usually manage mainstream schooling up to 12 years old or Primary 6 (6th grade); they should be able to live independently as an adult.
- IQ 40–55 Moderate Limited support. These individuals may not be able to reach Primary 2 (2nd grade) of school, and as an adult, they can live independently but may need some support.
- IQ 20–40 Severe   Extensive support. These individuals cannot live independently and need considerable help.
- IQ <20   Profound   Pervasive. These individuals require the most help.

Using the level of IQ to match a person's ability to function is problematic, because it is not an accurate reflection of life skills. Rather than use the IQ score only to determine how well a person can look after themselves, it is better to look at it the other way round, and base one's assessment on how much support they will need.

How common is intellectual disability?[3]

The estimated worldwide prevalence of intellectual disability is between 1 and 3 per cent of the population. How does it compare with other childhood disorders? "(Singapore statistics)

- Hypertension   1 in 6
- Asthma   1 in 12
- Diabetes type 2   1 in 12
- Epilepsy   1 in 26–100

- **Intellectual disability**　　　**1 in 33–100**
- Infant mortality ratio　　　1 in 166 live births
- Autism spectrum disorder　1 in 150
- Cerebral palsy　　　　　　1 in 200–300
- Childhood cancer (all)　　　1 in 333
- Down Syndrome　　　　　　1 in 800

Causes

The brain is our supreme command centre which controls our thoughts, memories, speech, the movement of our limbs, and the function of many organs inside our body.

Intellectual disability is thought to be the result of miswiring or atrophy of the nerves in the central nervous system. This results in slowing down or even stopping neural signals in their tracks.

Damage to the young brain can occur before, during, or after birth. We divide the causes into two major categories: genetics and environment. We realise that these two divisions may not be totally isolated from each other, and they can interact with one another. To this day, unfortunately, there are still people with intellectual disabilities where we cannot fathom the cause.

Genetic causes[7]

Genetic causes include chromosomal abnormalities, inborn errors of metabolism, random gene mutations and epigenetic conditions. There are literally hundreds of genetic causes, and these are listed in the references. The commonest chromosomal abnormality associated with intellectual disability is Down Syndrome. Gene mutations are also found in other syndromes like William Syndrome, Prader-Willi Syndrome, Fragile-X Syndrome, Rett Syndrome, just to name a few.

What is the link between genetics and brain development?

Genes control protein synthesis. All cells, including nerve cells, are made of proteins. The function of cells are controlled by enzymes and other proteins. Hence, genetic mutations of brain cells can result in abnormal protein production, thereby potentially affecting the structure and function of the brain.

(a) Brain malformation affecting the structure of the brain
    Microcephaly (small head) restricts the development of neurons
    Macrocephaly (big head)
    Abnormalities in brain architecture e.g. Lissencephaly
    Agenesis (absence) of the corpus callosum
(b) Disruptions in cellular metabolism with anomalies in the manufacturing and regulation of molecules essential to the brain and nerves
    Insufficient transport of necessary substances inside the cell
    Inadequate protein formation (gene transcription and translation)
    Lack of energetic substrates for the cell (mitochondria)
    Accumulation of toxic substances
(c) Abnormalities affecting the ability of neurons (the main brain cell population transporting information) to connect with each other: brain plasticity
    Brain plasticity is essential to acquire new skills through the many connections between neurons as experienced and stimulated by the environment.
    When cerebral plasticity is impaired, brain functions are restricted, resulting in altered information processing, inappropriate emotions and language difficulties, and making it difficult for the person to adapt to the environment.
    At the same time, the brain becomes more excitable and less able to filter information to protect itself from sensory over-stimulation and strong emotions.

In addition to intellectual disability, other disorders may accompany the intellectual delay:

    Language disorders
    Learning delays
    Emotional control difficulties
    Motor disorders

Epilepsy
Behavioural disorders
Sleep disorders
Eating disorders

Genetic defects may not be limited to neuronal cells; other organs like the heart, kidneys, eyes, may also be affected.

Environmental causes

Problems during pregnancy can affect the developing foetus, including lack of oxygen (hypoxia), maternal drugs, alcohol abuse, infections, etc. These can cause brain damage leading to intellectual disability.

Postnatal causes: jaundice, infections (meningitis, whooping cough), head trauma and other accidents, exposure to drugs and chemicals, and malnutrition, can affect brain development.

Investigations

A doctor needs to take a full medical history and do a physical examination including assessing development, doing a thorough neurological examination, and look for signs of thyroid hormone deficiency (hypothyroidism). The height, weight, head circumference and blood pressure must be measured.

Laboratory tests should include thyroid function, vitamin D level, full blood count, tests for congenital infections, and chromosome studies.

Magnetic resonance imaging or a computed tomographic scan can look inside the brain, and in some cases might help find the cause(s).

Therapy

We are able to help children achieve their maximum potential through more individualised education and several intervention therapies, including speech therapy, occupational therapy, physiotherapy, as well as music and art therapy. Should the individual display other disorders, such as epilepsy, ADHD, depression, sleep disturbances, etc., they should be treated appropriately.

Gene and CRISPR therapy[8]

There are some philosophical and ethical questions concerning manipulating a person's genes. We take a neutral stance here.

Gene mutations can cause developmental delays by producing
abnormal proteins which affect metabolic processes or nerve connections in
the brain. The burning question we are asking is whether we can or should
replace the defective or missing genes. We await an answer with bated
breath. But, looking at the successful introduction of gene therapy for other
genetic diseases like haemophilia, severe combined immunodeficiency and
retinitis pigmentosa, it might not be long before gene therapy becomes
available for neurodevelopmental conditions.

Dietary therapy

It has been observed that deficiency of vitamin D, vitamin B12, folic acid,
iodine, and severe iron deficiency is associated with impaired intellectual
function. Mental activity improves when these deficiencies are corrected.
We are already treating metabolic diseases like phenylketonuria and galac-
tosaemia by avoiding phenylalanine or milk. Other dietary manipulations
that have shown benefits include a ketogenic diet rich in fat plus non-syn-
thesised vitamins such as biotin or thiamine, or by providing a missing
enzyme with enzyme therapy.

Special education

Early intervention[9]

Early diagnosis of intellectual disability may allow for early intervention
though special education and behaviour therapy, and this has been shown
to maximise a child's potential. The class size should be kept as small as
possible so that the teacher-student ratio is maintained at an optimal
level. The training and therapy are best conducted by specially trained
teachers and therapists. The curriculum is holistic and inclusive, and the
pace of teaching is individualised, depending on the rate at which the
child progresses.

The areas covered in the early intervention programme include:

(a) Cognitive domain: Learning language, both verbal and written, handling numbers, mathematics calculations, problem-solving.
(b) Social and communication skills: This is conducted through direct interaction with the therapists and the student peers.
(c) Arts, music, sports: Students learn how to sing, dance, and play a musical instrument. They are taught drawing and painting, and play several sports including swimming.
(d) Behaviour guidance: If the child's behaviour is challenging (e.g. too aggressive or too passive), gentle modification is introduced.

Continuing education

In many countries, there is a trend for mildly intellectually disabled children to be integrated into regular mainstream nurseries, kindergartens, primary schools, secondary schools, and tertiary educational institutions. The more severely disabled will need to attend special schools where they receive multidisciplinary therapies. Most special schools take children up to the age of 18 years. Sheltered workshops provide training for outside employment for those in the late teens, but this may be limited in many countries.

Helping the family[10]

When parents are informed by the doctor that their child could be intellectually disabled, they may take the news badly, and either disbelieve the information, or become depressed. It is important for the doctor to be prepared for these responses. The parents might like to have a relative or friend to be present when the diagnosis is being presented. It is important to spend time to express what you, the parents feel, and if you do not believe the news, then either discuss with someone else or go back for another consultation. As parents you may want to seek a second opinion, and this should be expected. The doctor might take an understanding neutral approach, and perhaps adopt a slightly optimistic long-term forecast on how the child can improve with early intervention and treatment. Try to be positive and maintain some hope.

Conclusions

Intellectually challenged children are declining in numbers, thanks to preventive measures like rubella and other vaccinations, and better antenatal and birth management. Gene and CRISPR therapy is starting to show some promise in research but they are on the horizon for the future. Medicine can be used to treat some of the associated conditions, such as epilepsy, ADHD and depression. The backbone of therapy for these exceptional children is special education supplemented by multidisciplinary therapies. Intervention should be introduced as early as possible to maximise the child's potential. It is hoped that in time to come, these children can become more fully integrated into the mainstream education system. We should treat them as part of our family and take care of them from birth to departure.

References

1. Wikipedia. Intellectual disability. https://en.wikipedia.org/wiki/Intellectual_disability
2. Zeldin AS. Intellectual disability. Medscape 2021. https://emedicine.medscape.com/article/1180709-overview#showall
3. Special Olympics. Worldwide prevalence of intellectual disability. Special Olympics. https://www.specialolympics.org/about/intellectual-disabilities/what-is-intellectual-disability
4. Chow A. Psychometric & IQ testing. Annabelle Psychology. https://www.annabellepsychology.com/iq-testing
5. Oxford Learning. What's the score? Problems with IQ tests for kids. Oxford Learning 2015. https://www.oxfordlearning.com/whats-the-score-problems-with-iq-tests-for-kids/
6. Colmar S et al. Assessing intellectual disability in children: Are IQ measures sufficient, or even necessary? Australian Journal of Guidance & Counselling 2006; 16: 177–188. https://www.academia.edu/3130284/Assessing_Intellectual_Disability_in_Children_Are_IQ_Measures_Sufficient_or_Even_Necessary
7. Llyas M et al. The genetics of intellectual disability: advancing technology and gene editing. F1000Res 2020. https://www.ncbi.nlm.nih.gov/pmc/articles/PMC6966773/

8. Klein A. CRISPR has fixed the genetic cause of a learning disability. New Scientist 2018. https://www.newscientist.com/article/2161345-crispr-has-fixed-the-genetic-cause-of-a-learning-disability/
9. Early Intervention Foundation. What is early intervention? Early Intervention Foundation. https://www.eif.org.uk/why-it-matters/what-is-early-intervention
10. Sarvananthan R. Parenting a child with intellectual disability. Positive Parenting 2017. https://mypositiveparenting.org/2017/11/09/parenting-a-child-with-intellectual-disability/

14 Autism

Introduction

The spectrum of autism extends from the verbally fluent and slightly socially detached person at the mild end, to the nonverbal and socially isolated loner at the severe end. Some people on the mild end may not wish to be labelled autistic, and prefer to be viewed as "different". Children at the severe end, on the other hand, need a lot of help including early intervention, speech and occupational therapy, as well as long-term supportive care. To qualify for special education and to apply for financial help for expensive therapy, a diagnostic label is generally helpful. Many high-functioning autistic people are still insistent that we should not stick the label of autism on them. However, this is changing as they are becoming more accepted.

Definition[1-3]

Autism is a common but complex neurodevelopmental disorder characterised by early-onset difficulties in social communication and unusually restrictive repetitive behaviours and interests. It manifests as a wide spectrum, ranging from a mild hesitation in communicating with others, to someone who barely talks to anyone else. It encompasses the person who physically displays obsessionally recurring movements, to the savant with exceptionally gifted mathematics or artistic talents.

The early signs of autism are often subtle, but become clearer during the second and third year of life. The signs of autism are not transient, but rather persist over time. People do not grow out of autism, but some of the signs become less prominent. Autism is a lifelong condition.

Early signs

Early signs of autism include barely babbling, not using gestures such as pointing, and not responding to others by waving or nodding. Although poor eye contact is often listed as a feature of autistic children, this is an unreliable sign in Asians because they mostly have poor eye contact as part of Asian culture. They may display repetitive behaviours like flapping their hands or spinning the wheels of a toy car. They may pay more attention to objects than people, and although they can hear perfectly well, they may not respond when their name is called.

Diagnosis[4]

Before we can make a diagnosis of autism, an important question needs to be answered: "Is autism one condition, or is it several overlapping conditions?" Is it a single diagnosis or is it a composite of several diagnoses? The clinical presentation of autism is variable with a diversity of expressions, and therefore the diagnosis can be challenged or refuted. Without a definitive diagnosis, could we have misdiagnosed autism in some cases?

If we can link relevant and replicable investigations to the clinical manifestations, we can formulate a hypothesis of cause and effect. Unfortunately, at the moment, we have neither unequivocal clinical findings nor clearcut investigatory findings.

The problem is compounded by the fact that there is a myriad of diagnostic tools for autism, and there is no consensus which one of these tests is most accurate.

Classifying systems

- Diagnostic and Statistical Manual 5th revision (DSM-5)
- International Classification of Diseases 10th revision (ICD-10)

The DSM-5 and the ICD-10 are classifying systems, not diagnostic tests. They list the major components to consider, and they guide one towards thinking whether or not to refer someone for a more definitive diagnosis.

Diagnostic and statistical manual 5ᵗʰ edition (DSM-5)

The American Psychiatric Association introduced the Diagnostic and Statistical Manual to guide the classification of many psychiatric disorders, and it is now in its 5ᵗʰ edition. The DSM-5 lists two major areas that need to be present in order to consider someone with autism.

1. **Social communication and interaction deficits**
   The autistic individual prefers to be alone and there is little social reciprocity, They do not seem to want to share interests with others, and there can be verbal as well as nonverbal communication difficulties. There appear to be problems developing and maintaining friends. As they get older, they may have difficulty with small talk and reading facial expressions, which can make them seem insensitive. They may take what is said quite literally, for example when asked to "take a seat", they may pick up a seat and take it elsewhere.
2. **Restricted or repetitive behaviours, interests and activities**
   Children may line up toys in a ritualistic way, flapping hands, pacing up and down, imitating words or phrases repeatedly. They may be fixed on certain routines, preferring the same sequence of activities like dressing themselves and having breakfast before brushing their teeth. There can be restricted patterns of interests like having specific in-depth knowledge of astronomy or dinosaurs. Some individuals are distracted by background noise so they cannot focus on what is said by others.

Diagnostic tests[5]

To make a definitive diagnosis of autism, these are the following commonly used tests:

- Autism Diagnostic Interview
- Autism Diagnostic Observation Schedule
- Checklist for Autism in Toddlers
- Childhood Autism Rating Scale
- Gilliam Autism Rating Scale

It is uncertain which method is the most accurate because there has not been a large-scale trial comparing one method with another.

All diagnostic tests agree that autism is a spectrum disorder and varies significantly from person to person. The above descriptions may not be found in everyone. Some may require more, and others less support in their daily lives. A small percentage (probably 10 per cent or less) show special abilities in visual memory, art, music, maths and science.

Prevalence[6-8]

The prevalence of autism differs from one country to another, ranging from 1:59 in the US, to 1:150 in Singapore.

According to a 2021 report,[9] there has been a 787 per cent increase in the incidence of autism in England during the past two decades. However,

Table 14-1.　Prevalence of autism in different countries (WHO 2020)

Country	Prevalence
United States	1 in 59
Canada	1 in 66
Ireland	1 in 78
South Korea	1 in 91
Hong Kong	1 in 99
Saudi Arabia	1 in 99
India	1 in 113
China	1 in 125
England	1 in 128
Japan	1 in 128
Thailand	1 in 128
Taiwan	1 in 129
Russia	1 in 130
Germany	1 in 138
France	1 in 144
Australia	1 in 150
Singapore	1 in 150

the authors do not think this is a real increase in the number of cases, but rather an increase in the number of cases diagnosed due to heightened awareness of the condition.

Associated conditions[10]

Another confounding factor is that some autistic persons may have other associated conditions. Some 30 per cent will have intellectual disability, over 30 per cent have attention deficit hyperactivity disorder (ADHD) and between 10 and 20 per cent will have epilepsy. Other associated diagnoses include obsessive-compulsive disorder (OCD), and gastrointestinal disorders. Clinically, it is important to decide whether or not these comorbidities should be viewed as part of the autistic diagnostic spectrum, or whether they should be classified as additional separate diagnoses. Paediatricians tend to take the latter route and separate autism from the other comorbidities, and this appears to be the current consensus.

Are boys more likely to be autistic?

Another finding that also needs to be explained is the apparent predominance of males diagnosed with autism. There are several publications suggesting that boys are five times or more likely to be diagnosed with autism than girls. However, recent studies suggest that the diagnosis of autism in girls is frequently missed because they display less repetitive behaviours, their restricted range of interests tend to be considered as normal for girls, and the assessors have less issues with smaller vocabulary and delayed learning. Most current researchers assert that in the community, the male:female ratio is about equal.

Causes[11]

Autism has a myriad of causes. Trying to disentangle the causes of autism is like finding one's way through a dense forest with only the guide of a global positioning system, which sets the general direction you want to travel, but does not help you overcome the obstacles that can block your progress.

Because autism is a complex disorder, there are potentially many causes.[1] We can stratify the causes into several layers. The basic layer is the underlying genetic and environmental causes which will interact with one another. The genes will express themselves in many ways, including biochemically and neurodevelopmentally. The next layer to explore is the brain: How its structure, neurocircuitry, and function of the brain modulate behaviour. Environmental influences are still pervasive, and can alter a child's behaviour before or after birth. The factors potentially affecting foetal or child development are numerous, and may include diet, maternal-foetal or postnatal infections, toxins, etc. They may even occur together and cause autism.

It is difficult to pin down which aetiology is the dominant one. To date, there are no indisputable scientific experiments, no incontrovertible imaging or genetic findings that can pinpoint the main causes. For example, genetic probes which are the most promising research findings, have led to the discovery of hundreds of possible genes linked to autism. It is confusing. But complexity itself does not negate that one is on the right track. It just makes it harder to prove the aetiology or aetiologies.

Genetic causes[12–14]

Why are genes thought to be linked to autism? It originates from the famous studies of identical and non-identical twins. When one twin has autism, then an identical twin has a 60 to 90 per cent chance of developing it. In contrast, a nonidentical or fraternal twin of the same sex only shares the autistic diagnosis around 30 per cent of the time, and different sex (boy-girl) twin pairs share the diagnosis 20 per cent of the time. The concordance rate for different-aged siblings is about 10 per cent, while the general population risk ranges from 0.5 to 1.8 per cent depending on which country is surveyed.

The fact that the identical twin concordance rate is not 100 per cent suggests that there must be other factors involved, most probably environmental.

Hunt for variants or mutations

Humans match each other quite closely, with 99.9 per cent of the order of their base pair DNAs identical with one another. The non-identical 0.1 per cent are known as variants and are either nonfunctional, or may contribute to disease risk, or may even protect one from diseases. Gene variants arise from mutations. Nowadays, the terms variants and mutations are used interchangeably.

Are variants or mutations inheritable? Yes and no. Some variants can cause inheritable diseases, like those associated with autism. Fortunately, they are relatively rare.

De novo variants[15]

De novo or brand new variations of the genes are usually thought to arise spontaneously and quite passively. Most do not cause any problems, but sometimes, they can result in serious diseases, including autism. Some spontaneous mutations may occur in either the sperm or the ovum before or after fertilisation. While these germ-line mutations were not inherited from earlier generations, they can affect the offspring and future generations.

Whole exome sequencing (WES)[16]

Thanks to the human genome project, an international scientific research project that identified and mapped out all the base pairs or genes that make up human DNA, we can try to map out the genes for autism.

The human genome consists of three billion nucleotides or "letters" of DNA, but only 1.5 per cent of these letters can be responsible for protein synthesis. These protein-synthesising nucleotides are known as "exomes".

The search for the entire protein-manufacturing exomes is known as WES. This procedure has revolutionised the study of genes in autism. Using this new technology, scientists can look at all 21,000 genes comprising 180,000 exome nucleotides, which constitute a miniscule fraction of the three billion base pairs of the entire human genome.

Several hundreds of gene variations have been found in autistic subjects. When researchers looked at the function of these genes, they were able to group them by their different functions. One group of variants was involved in the neurons, influencing the neuronal cell adhesion molecules, and thereby affecting the function of nerves. Another group of variants affected the ubiquitin pathway which helps in the synthesis of new proteins, and the destruction of defective proteins.

With current whole exome sequencing, we can explore all the exome genes at the same time, which not only widens the search, but simultaneously cuts down the time taken for research. These are exciting times, and hopefully in future, we can identify the more important genes associated with autism, and perhaps lead to prevention and treatment.

Neurological causes

Brain pathophysiology[17–23]

Exploring the genetics is only the first step in our attempts to understand the causes of autism. The next step is to understand the neuroanatomy and the neurophysiology of the autistic brain and how it differs from the non-autistic brain. Fortunately, there have been recent major advances in mapping out the form and function of the brain and the nerve connections.

The brain has billions of nerve cells or neurons. However, in autism, these neurons are not communicating with one another properly. Researchers are trying to pinpoint which parts of the brain are affected, and the mechanisms of the problems found in autism. Older studies using electroencephalography (EEG) showed increased prevalence of epilepsy in autistic subjects, but the use of simple resting state EEG has inconsistent results.

One major advance in understanding the function of the brain is the development of functional magnetic resonance imaging. This detects increased oxygen that is supplied to active brain nerve cells. Compared to non-autistic subjects, autistic individuals have reduced activities in certain areas of the brain, namely the superior temporal sulcus and amygdala, and this is thought to be due to reduced neuronal connectivity.

Other imaging techniques, including diffusion tensor imaging which detects the flow of water along the white matter, and magnetic resonance spectroscopy which detects the neurotransmitters glutamate and Gamma-AminoBenzoic Acid. They have led to new findings, but their significance and therapeutic applications are not conclusive, and further research is needed.

Conditions associated with autism[24–27]

Autistic individuals frequently have other conditions, and this can often complicate matters either by delaying the diagnosis of autism, or being treated with medicines that bring out other symptoms because of the side effects. These associated conditions need to be treated separately.

- ADHD
- Epilepsy
- Irritability, Aggressive Behaviour, Temper Tantrums, Self-Injuries
- Anxiety, Depression
- Sleep Disturbances

Management of autism[28]

What are the main targets for management?

The main targets for therapy are to improve communication and social skills, promote academic functioning, decrease negative behaviour, and ultimately improve the quality of life of the autistic individual.

The proven ways of achieving most of these goals are through special education with trained teachers and therapists in a small class, preferably starting early in the child's life. The interventions include occupational therapy, physiotherapy, social skills training, speech and language therapy, and the use of music, art and sports to enhance the various forms of therapy.

Is there a dichotomy between medical and non-medical therapy? Meaning, should medical therapy be relegated only to comorbid conditions associated with autism? Or should we combine special education and behavioural intervention strategies with medicine?

The answer must be "yes". One can indeed combine the different therapy modalities. Ideally, all intervention strategies should be evidence-based. Trials are still ongoing comparing the different treatments of autism, and in reality, many parents are impatient and will embark on different forms of therapy in the hope that some will be of benefit.

Medical treatment

Currently, no medicine has been proven to significantly improve the core symptoms of autism, namely the communication socialising difficulties, and the restrictive repetitive movements. Medicine can help with some of the associated manifestations of autism, which include ADHD, OCD, epilepsy, aggressive and self-injurious behaviour, anxiety, and some abdominal symptoms.

Medicine and diets that do not work

There are no large double-blind placebo-controlled trials for the treatments and medicine listed below. However, many parents believe that they work. Provided they do not do any harm, and are not prohibitively expensive or time-consuming, and if they do not displace therapy that is proven to work, then it is probably all right for parents and patients to continue with the therapy below. Personally, I would not recommend their use.

- Anti-Fungal and Anti-Yeast Medication
- Cannabis and Marijuana
- Chelation Therapy
- Complementary Alternative Medicine
- Trans-craniosacral Magnetic Stimulation
- Faecal Microbial Transplantation
- Herbs and Homeopathic Treatments
- Hyperbaric Oxygen Therapy
- Neurofeedback Therapy
- Secretin
- Special Diets (Gluten or casein-free, sugar free)
- High dose vitamins (B vitamins, E vitamin, folic acid, etc)
- Supplement Therapy (Omega 3 Fatty Acids)

Early intervention[29-32]

Currently the most important avenue for managing autism is by early intervention, starting at two years of age or younger. There are several techniques, but they are based on behavioural therapy, using rewards to encourage doing specific activities, and not using punishment. The teaching is individualised, follows a structured timetable, and the child is taught in a quiet environment. On top of these treatments are additional speech and communication therapy, occupational therapy, physical therapy, as well as art and music therapy.

There is a strong emphasis in using visual cues as instructions. For example, a "posting exercise" begins by asking a child to "post" or insert some coins into a plastic container with a slot for the coins. When that is accomplished, the child is praised, and then given a two-part task in which a miniature toy is first inserted into a small transparent plastic ball with a hinged opening. Once the miniature toy is inserted into the plastic ball, the second part is to take the transparent ball and "post" or insert it into an even larger container with a large round opening. On completion of this second phase, the child is again complimented and either given another more complex "posting" task, or given another unrelated activity. At the end of a series of tasks, the child can be rewarded with a sticker.

The daily timetable is presented visually with separate pictures illustrating each task drawn onto removable stickers. Once the task is completed, the sticker of that activity is removed from the timetable and placed into a "completed" container.

The teaching is labour intensive because of the low student to teacher ratio. The advantage is that the teacher can discover which activities the child enjoys most, and this is used to start off the programme. The student is closely monitored, given a lot of verbal encouragement, and if appropriate, the child is initially shown how to do the task. Time devoted to each activity is structured and adhered to. The teacher should engage the student, speak literally and avoid metaphors and abstract words. Wherever possible, they should aim to reduce the extra stressors on the child, and to remove sensory distractions like loud sounds and bright lights.

Guided by the above principles, the activities chosen can range very widely from teaching language by story-telling, matching words, using or making objects to match the pictures in a book, or singing a song or dancing to supplement parts of the story.

Should we correct behavioural differences?

There are two schools of thought on how to alter an autistic person's behaviour, especially if it is seen to be rather unconventional, like prolonged flapping of the hands, head-shaking, pacing up and down, or making grunting or shouting sounds. The inclusive school believes that we should do nothing and accept this behaviour as normal but different. The conventional school believes that the behaviours listed above should be modified.

If you want to take the conventional route, then there are two major methods used: behavioural therapy and cognitive therapy, or a combination of the two.

The primary focus of behaviour therapy is to change the way an autistic individual responds to other people or to the current situation. For example, if a person is flapping incessantly, then they are gently told to stop, and if they stop, they may be rewarded by being thanked, or given a raisin.

In contrast, cognitive therapy is to change the way the person thinks about a situation. For example, if the person is afraid to enter a room, then they are taught to take some relaxation exercises like deep breathing, and to think of something more soothing.

Practical advice on how parents and caregivers can cope with their autistic child[33-35]

Just as there is a spectrum of autistic individuals, there is also a spectrum of families into which they belong. Some families are thrown out of balance when they are challenged with a child who needs extra support and management. Others cope with the myriad of difficulties with self-assurance. Here we will focus on the more severe end of the autistic spectrum that poses stresses upon their families. What are the challenges facing them and how do we address them? Below are some frequently asked questions:

1. **How can we come to terms with the diagnosis?**
   It can come as a shock to learn that your child has autism. No amount of groundwork can prepare you for this. You might go through a wide range of emotions ranging from fear to anxiety and despair. We love our children so much, and we want to give them the very best in life, but now we fear the worst. You may deny the diagnosis initially, and later, you might become angry and even depressed, before finally beginning to accept the diagnosis. Some of your friends may try to convince you that autism is not a disease, but merely a different condition that will sort itself out in the end. But this will probably not alleviate your grief.

It is important to try to obtain more information, either through online sites, books, or talking to recognised teachers, psychologists or medical specialists about the diagnosis. Given the complexity of autism, it is important that you and your family seek professional advice early, as this can help you learn how to engage and connect with your child, and to become more flexible and understanding of your child's behaviour, feelings, and development.

2. **How should we deal with other family members' reactions to the diagnosis?**

   You may have begun to accept the diagnosis of your child, but now you have to inform other members of your family. Each one will probably respond differently. Perhaps you might want to talk to each member separately, including your spouse, siblings, grandparents, and other caregivers. The reason is that autism is a lifelong condition that requires teamwork and long-term management. This can only come about when everybody accepts and understands the condition and learns how to work together to cope.

   Having a child with autism can be very lonely for you. It is not uncommon for parents to keep the child's diagnosis hidden from their immediate family and even their friends and colleagues. It is probably better not to conceal your child's condition from others, because eventually you might need to enlist the help of your friends, neighbours and other members of the community.

3. **How should we treat our autistic child?**

   Accept your child as they are. Accept their idiosyncrasies, their unusual mannerisms, their quirks. There are times they will be exasperating, like crying for long periods, and nothing you do will stop the crying. Don't give up. Engage them, love them. Children will grow up and change with time. You too will learn to adapt.

4. **How should we change the physical environment of our home?**

   Autistic children are sensitive to the environment. First, the home environment should be safe. Avoid getting furniture with sharp corners. Keep dangerous implements away. Cover electric sockets with electric plug protectors. Construct window grilles to prevent any accidental falls.

   Reduce noise because many autistic individuals have sensitive hearing and cannot stand loud noise. This also applies to television, radio, mobile devices and home cinemas. They put their hands over their ears. This is the same with lights: avoid bright lights. Many autistic people do not tolerate glaring lights and they cover their eyes.

It would also be useful to have a variety of safe toys. Some autistic children like to line up objects, like cars, so perhaps one should not buy too many similar vehicles.

5. **Should we set a timetable?**

Yes, autistic children learn and develop better with a predictable programme. You should set up a detailed structured schedule that can be followed every day. This includes waking up at around the same time, brushing teeth, washing face, toileting, changing clothes, having breakfast, playtime, exercise time, etc., all the way to bedtime.

6. **How should we communicate with our child?**

Some autistic children may have delayed speech, and some remain silent for much of their lives. Look out for subtle nonverbal cues and facial expressions which can be reduced in autistic individuals. They may have decreased movements so it can sometimes be difficult to read their body language, facial gestures, as well as their responses to food, toys, and other people. If they are not looking at you, turn their head to focus on your face. Use a combination of visual and auditory clues to communicate, supplemented by supplying the words to describe the activities or objects.

Try not to spend too much time watching television, playing with mobile phones or laptop computers. Sure, you can allow some online activities, but this should not preclude human interactions, going outside to explore the world, and other pursuits. Anecdotal evidence suggests that online activities do not stimulate communication or speech. Early intervention programmes will include speech and communication therapy.

7. **How to optimize learning**

Find out their strengths and weaknesses. What do they enjoy? Do they enjoy certain activities like drawing, playing the piano, or constructing objects with building blocks? Make playtime fun, but limit the time devoted to any particular activity, so it does not become obsessional.

8. **How to tackle undesired behaviours**

Some autistic children indulge in prolonged repetitive behaviours, like clapping, flapping hands, rocking, and even self-injurious activities.

They may make unusually loud noises or scream continuously. One approach is to distract them and try to persuade them to take part in another activity or play with another toy. Try to discover if there may be some recognisable triggers for these behaviours. For example, is it in response to your refusal to give them what they want? Maybe you do not realise what they really want, and they are unable to express themselves in words, choosing instead to scream.

In the case of self-injurious or dangerous behaviours like head-banging, biting, pushing, or scratching, you need to stop these activities immediately. If necessary, make an appointment to consult a doctor.

9. **Should we engage in special therapy?**

These include speech and communication therapy, occupational therapy, physical therapy, music and art therapy. Most special schools, nurseries and kindergartens with a focus on autistic children, should be able to provide some of these forms of therapy. When you have identified areas that you think your child might need extra encouragement and help with, then you might like to discuss if they are really beneficial, and where to find these forms of therapy.

10. **What will our autistic child's future look like, and how should we cope?**

Different stages of the autistic individual's life will require different approaches. The young autistic child may need early intervention centres that may help in several ways, including providing family support, speech therapy, occupational therapy, and special education. Opportunities for socialising needs to be organised, so that the child can mix with other children, be given opportunities to engage in art, music, sports, and outdoor activities. The long-term future may require drawing up a will, and setting aside some funds in the event that the individuals are unable to take care of themselves, especially after the parents have passed on.

11. **How can we avoid being overwhelmed by too much information on the Internet?**

As parents, you might be googling the Internet to search for as much information as you can about autism. Indeed, cyberspace has a vast storehouse of material in text and videos. But you might be overwhelmed by too much information, some of which may be inaccurate. So, it is important for you to verify the reliability of what you have read.

You should also discuss what you have found with other professionals to evaluate its accuracy and relevance.

12. **How do we cope with the strain on our marriage?**

Looking after an autistic child can be a heavy strain on one's marriage. Sometimes, getting relatives and friends to help out can alleviate the problem. If not, one may have to look for marital or family counselling for help.

13. **Who would be best to confirm a diagnosis of autism?**

The diagnosis of autism spectrum disorder should be made by an experienced physician, paediatrician, psychiatrist, or psychologist familiar with autism. A teacher, counsellor, or another parent, should also be able to guide you. You can also search the Internet for websites that can lead you to resource centres, special schools, and government websites dealing with autism. These websites might be able to provide information and advice, and direct you to the appropriate psychologists and medical specialists to obtain a diagnosis.

There are several centres that can help. In Singapore, the Autism Resource Centre (ARC) was set up specifically to focus on the education of autism for families and autistic individuals. ARC has also been running Certificate and Diploma in Autism courses for educators from both mainstream and special education institutions. They also run parent training workshops for parents and the public. The Rainbow Centre also provides family services in Singapore.

14. **Which preschools and schools to choose from?**

There are several factors to consider. This includes where on the autistic spectrum your child falls into. Are there any co-morbid problems, like ADHD, epilepsy, aggressive behaviours? How far is the school from where you live, and is transport provided? It's best to visit the schools and discuss your child with the teachers, principals and other parents.

15. **We are finding it hard to cope financially. Where can we find help?**

Some children with autism require special education, early intervention, and other forms of therapy, but these can be quite costly. What kind of help is available for low-income families who are raising children with autism? Fortunately, there are government organisations and charitable foundations that can give a helping hand. See resources on page 161.

16. What are the myths associated with autism?

- Autistic people do not show empathy: Actually, they can and do show empathy for others.
- They do not wish to make friends with others: Their difficulties making friends should not be interpreted as a lack of desire to have friends.
- They all have special talents: Less than 10 per cent have savant skills like calculations, puzzles, drawing or music.
- They have zero sense of humour: They may display their sense of humour in different and more subtle ways.
- They cannot have romantic relationships: Some are capable of having such associations.
- They are intellectually disabled: Yes, many do not score well on IQ tests, but not all. Because part of the IQ tests is timed, some autistic people get stuck on one question; it is therefore necessary to assess their intelligence in other ways.
- All autistic individuals are alike: Every person on the autistic spectrum is different; they have their own unique talents and personality, and challenges.

Future challenges

Hopes for the future include the following:

(a) **Prevention**

Prevention is better than cure. If we can discover the causes of childhood developmental conditions, we may be able to prevent more of these states. In fact, the incidence of Down Syndrome and cerebral palsy has fallen, and I hope that autism will follow suit. Whole genome sequencing during pregnancy or at birth may lead to earlier identification of autism before or shortly after birth, which can potentially lead to some form of intervention or therapy to correct biochemical deficiencies. Advances in gene therapy or genome editing (such as CRISPR) may one day correct mutations for some genes as well.

(b) **Inclusive Education**

Different, not disabled. I do not believe in segregating children with differences into separate schools or institutions. Children have different abilities and interests, but we should not partition them into isolated schools. They can still join in other activities such as sports, art, music, dance, etc. We need to develop a mindset that we are all part of a family.

Better understanding of the neurophysiology of autism can help us better understand human neurodiversity, and how each of us has our own unique brain connectivity and functions.

(c) **New Technologies**

Creating new technologies to help the disabled should be given more funding. Enhancing communication, employing artificial intelligence, facilitating the integration of special children into society, and helping them to travel or shop by themselves can be developed further.

(d) **Stem Cells**

Stem cells may one day be developed to produce different types of cells, either to replace neurons affected by autism, or to do research into drugs or toxins that can influence these autism-simulated stem cell neurons.

(e) **Dark Matter**

We are currently looking at the protein-related exome genes which comprises only 1 per cent of all our genes. We have barely started looking at the "dark matter" non-protein related intron genes. Like the dark matter in the universe, we have a long way to go, but we may be surprised by what this research might lead to.

(f) **Infant Brain Imaging Studies**

Ongoing studies using conventional magnetic resonance imaging (MRI) scans, coupled with EEG and eye tracking tests, are being used to help in the early diagnosis of young autistic children between six months and two years old. These children are also being followed up with repeated MRI scans and psychological tests to monitor the efficacy of special education, the different forms of therapy, and medicine. The objective is to see if there are any early structural changes in the brain of children that can detect autism earlier, and which hopefully can lead to earlier intervention.

Conclusions

Teamwork is the foundation of coping with autism. The good news is that there are now quite a number of organisations, schools, psychological and medical services that can help. The problem is trying to find what would be best for your child and for your family. The Internet can overwhelm you with too much information, and the most attractive site may not offer the best advice or therapy. Discuss it with as many people as possible, including teachers, psychologists, doctors, and other parents.

Autism is a challenge at many levels. Educationally, it requires us to reduce class size and to individualise the curriculum and pace of instruction, and to employ positive rather than negative methods of teaching. It affects families and caregivers, requiring them to adapt their child's physical environment and activities, and to plan for the long term. Some individuals on the more severe end of the autism spectrum may need lifelong support and care. This may require intervention from the state to plan for the long term. Philosophically, autism forces us to rethink whether we should label people on the spectrum as disabled, disadvantaged, exceptional, or differently able. Currently there is a movement to remove high-functioning autistic individuals from being labeled as autistic, and to consider them as normal. Ideally, in the long run, we want an inclusive society that does not discriminate against anyone.

References

1. Frith U. Autism: A Very Short Introduction. Oxford University Press 2008. ISBN: 978-0-19-920756-5
2. Fletcher-Watson S & Happé F. Autism: A New Introduction to Psychological Theory and Current Debate. Routledge 2019. ISBN: 978-1-138-10612-3.
3. Casanova EL & Casanova MF. Defining autism: a guide to brain, biology, and behavior. Jessica Kingsley Publishers 2019. ISBN: 978-1-78592-722-5.
4. Gallo DP. Diagnosing autism spectrum disorders. Wiley-Blackwell 2010. ISBN: 978-0-470-74923-4.
5. ABA Centers of America. How Is Autism Diagnosed? Screening, Testing and Diagnosis. ABA Centers of America. https://www.abacenters.com/how-is-autism-diagnosed-screening-testing-and-diagnosis/
6. World Health Organisation. Autism https://www.who.int/news-room/fact-sheets/detail/autism-spectrum-disorders
7. Russell G et al. Time trends in autism diagnosis over 20 years: a UK population-based cohort study. The Journal of Child Psychology and Psychiatry 2021. https://acamh.onlinelibrary.wiley.com/doi/10.1111/jcpp.13505

8. Wikipedia. Epidemiology of autism. https://en.wikipedia.org/wiki/Epidemiology_of_autism
9. University of Exeter. Number diagnosed with autism jumps 787 percent in two decades. Medical Xpress. https://medicalxpress.com/news/2021-09-autism-cent-decades.html
10. Furfaro H. Conditions that accompany autism, explained. Spectrum News 2018. https://www.spectrumnews.org/news/conditions-accompany-autism-explained/
11. Wikipedia. Causes of autism. https://en.wikipedia.org/wiki/Causes_of_autism
12. Hadley D. Genetics of autism spectrum disorders. eMedicine 2022. https://emedicine.medscape.com/article/2024885-overview
13. Sarris M. Twins study finds large genetic influence in autism. Interactive Autism Network 2014. https://iancommunity.org/autism-twins-study
14. Zeliadt M. Autism genetics, explained. Spectrum News 2021. https://www.spectrumnews.org/news/autism-genetics-explained/
15. Alonso-Gonzalez A et al. A. De novo Mutations (DNMs) in Autism Spectrum Disorder (ASD): Pathway and Network Analysis. Frontiers in Genetics 2018. https://www.frontiersin.org/articles/10.3389/fgene.2018.00406/full
16. Yu TW et al. Using whole exome sequencing to identify the causes of autism. Neurone 2013; 77: 259–273. https://www.ncbi.nlm.nih.gov/pmc/articles/PMC3694430/
17. Brasic JR. Pathophysiology of autism spectrum disorder. Medscape 2021. https://emedicine.medscape.com/article/912781-overview#a3
18. Gabrielsen TP et al. Functional MRI (fMRI) connectivity in children with autism. Molecular Autism 2018; 9: 67. https://molecularautism.biomedcentral.com/articles/10.1186/s13229-018-0248-y
19. Lau WKW et al. Resting state (fMRI) abnormalities in autism spectrum disorders. Nature News 2019; 9: 3892. https://www.nature.com/articles/s41598-019-40427-7
20. Solso S. Diffusion tensor imaging MRI in autism spectrum disorder toddlers. Biological Psychiatry 2016; 79: 676–684. https://www.sciencedirect.com/science/article/pii/S0006322315005697
21. Ford TC & Crewther DP. A comprehensive review of the magnetic resonance spectroscopy (H-MRS) in autism spectrum disorder. Frontiers in Molecular Neuroscience 2016. https://www.frontiersin.org/articles/10.3389/fnmol.2016.00014/full
22. Bosl WJ et al. EEG analytics for early detection of autism spectrum disorder. Scientific Reports 2018. https://www.nature.com/articles/s41598-018-24318-x

23. Wang J *et al.* Resting state EEG abnormalities in autism spectrum disorders. Journal of Neurodevelopmental Disorders 2013; 5: 24. https://jneurodevdisorders.biomedcentral.com/articles/10.1186/1866-1955-5-24

24. National Fragile X Foundation. Fragile-X and autism. National Fragile X Foundation https://fragilex.org/understanding-fragile-x/fragile-x-syndrome/autism/

25. Jeste SS. Tuberous Sclerosis Complex (TSC) and autism spectrum disorders. TSC Alliance 2013. https://www.tscalliance.org/about-tsc/signs-and-symptoms-of-tsc/brain-and-neurological-function/tsc-and-autism-spectrum-disorders/

26. Deweerdt S. Rett Syndrome's link to autism, explained. Spectrum News 2019. https://www.spectrumnews.org/news/rett-syndromes-link-to-autism-explained/

27. Oberman LM *et al.* Autism spectrum disorder in Phelan-McDermid Syndrome. Orphanet Journal of Rare Diseases 2015. https://ojrd.biomedcentral.com/articles/10.1186/s13023-015-0323-9

28. Chedd N & Levine K. Treatment planning for children with autism spectrum disorders. John Wiley & Sons Inc 2013. ISBN: 978-0-470-88223-8.

29. National Institute of Child Health and Human Development. What are the treatments for autism? National Institute of Child Health and Human Development. https://www.nichd.nih.gov/health/topics/autism/conditioninfo/treatments

30. Gordon D. Seeing the benefits of early intervention in autism. Brain & Life 2009. https://www.brainandlife.org/articles/early-intervention-in-autism/

31. Tsang LPM *et al.* Autism spectrum disorder: early identification and management in primary care (Singapore). Singapore Medical Journal 2019. http://www.smj.org.sg/article/autism-spectrum-disorder-early-identification-and-management-primary-care

32. Cherney K & Seladi-Schulman J. Everything You Need to Know About Autism Spectrum Disorder (ASD). Healthline 2021. https://www.healthline.com/health/autism

Resources

Singapore Autism Resource Centre. https://www.autism.org.sg/
Singapore Rainbow Centre. https://www.rainbowcentre.org.sg/
Singapore St Andrew's Autism Centre. https://www.saac.org.sg/
Malaysia Autism Link. https://www.autism.my/

Malacca Malaysia. http://www.wingsmelaka.org.my/
Australia Autism Spectrum. https://www.autismspectrum.org.au/
UK National Autistic Society. https://www.autism.org.uk/

Online Books and Courses

Infobooks. 15+ Free Autism Books
https://www.infobooks.org/free-pdf-books/psychology/autism/

Infiniteach. Free Autism Resources
https://free.infiniteach.com/autism-resources/

Special Learning House 2021
https://www.speciallearninghouse.com/

Autism Society Resources
https://autismsociety.org/resources-by-topic/

15 Attention deficit hyperactivity disorder (ADHD)

Introduction[1,2]

Most of us have some symptoms that fit into the diagnosis of ADHD. If you cannot sit still, keep fidgeting with your fingers, your mind wanders, and you cannot pay sufficient attention to finish what you are doing, then you might have ADHD. Hands up those of you who have these symptoms!

Difficulties with diagnosis

The problem with making a diagnosis of ADHD is that it is a spectrum, and the boundary between normal and abnormal is blurred. There are no laboratory or brain imaging studies that are consistently diagnostic. Therefore, we rely almost exclusively on a constellation of symptoms and signs.

Children who present only with inattention without physical hyperactivity, are often missed or their diagnosis delayed, especially in girls. It is only when school exam results come back below expectations, or teachers complain to the parents that their child is daydreaming, that the problem surfaces.

Paradoxically, children who are physically hyperactive and impulsive, might also be missed especially the boys, because it is assumed that it is natural for them to be energetic, aggressive and talkative. It is only the extreme end of the spectrum where the student is excessively boisterous, loses his temper, injures someone else, or is at risk of being expelled from the preschool or school, that parents seek medical or psychological help.

The diagnostic and statistical manual 5th edition (DSM-5)[3]

The American Psychiatric Association's Diagnostic and Statistical Manual 5th Edition (DSM-5)[3] is helpful in classifying the system but it is not a diagnostic test. It divides ADHD into two categories:

(a) Inattentive Type (used to be called Attention Deficit Disorder or ADD), and

(b) Hyperactivity and Impulsive Type (ADHD).

(a) **Inattentive type (ADD)**

You need six (or five for people over 17 years) of the following symptoms that occur frequently, have lasted for more than six months, and found in at least two settings (e.g. school and home):

- Has problems staying focused on tasks or activities, such as during lectures, conversations or long reading.
- Does not pay close attention to details, or makes careless mistakes in school or job tasks.
- Does not seem to listen when spoken to (i.e. seems to be somewhere else).
- Does not follow through on instructions and does not complete schoolwork, chores or job duties (may start tasks but quickly loses focus).
- Has problems organising tasks and work (for instance, does not manage time well; has messy, disorganized work; misses deadlines).
- Avoids or dislikes tasks that require sustained mental effort, such as preparing reports and completing forms.
- Often loses things needed for tasks or daily life, such as school papers, books, keys, wallet, mobile phone and eyeglasses.
- Is easily distracted.
- Forgets daily tasks, such as doing chores and running errands. Older teens and adults may forget to return phone calls, pay bills and keep appointments.

(b) **Hyperactive and Impulsive type (ADHD)**

You need six (or five for people over 17 years) of the following symptoms that occur frequently, have lasted for more than 6 months, and found in at least two settings (e.g. school and home):

- Fidgets with or taps hands or feet, or squirms in the seat.
- Not able to stay seated (in classroom, workplace).

- Runs about or climbs where it is inappropriate.
- Unable to play or do leisure activities quietly.
- Always "on the go", as if driven by a motor.
- Talks too much.
- Blurts out an answer before a question is completed (for instance, may complete someone else's sentences, cannot wait and barges in inappropriately during a conversation).
- Has difficulty waiting his or her turn, such as while waiting in line.
- Interrupts or intrudes on others (for instance, cuts into another person's game or activity, or starts using other people's things without permission). Older teens and adults may take over what others are doing, without permission.

ADHD tests[4]

Doctors, psychologists and educationalists can use one of the following rating scales to help them diagnose and track ADHD symptoms. Examples of diagnostic tests include the following:

- **The Test of Variables of Attention.**[5] This is a computerised, objective measure of attention and inhibitory control for four years old and above.
- **The Vanderbilt Assessment Scale.**[6] This 55-question assessment tool reviews symptoms of ADHD. It also looks for other conditions such as conduct disorder, oppositional-defiant disorder, anxiety, and depression.
- **The Child Attention Profile.** This scale is generally filled out by teachers and tracks common ADHD symptoms.
- **Behaviour Assessment System for Children.** This test looks for things like hyperactivity, aggression, and conduct problems. It also looks for anxiety, depression, attention and learning problems, and lack of certain essential skills.
- **Child Behaviour Checklist/Teacher Report Form.** Among other things, this scale looks at physical complaints, aggressive or delinquent behaviour, and withdrawal symptoms.
- **Conners Rating Scale.** This is a questionnaire that asks about aspects such as behaviour, work, school studies, and social life. They can show how these symptoms affect areas like grades, job, home life, and relationships.

Differential diagnosis[7]

It is important to differentiate ADHD from conditions whose symptoms overlap. This includes an overactive thyroid or thyrotoxicosis, where there can be inattention and hyperactivity. Some children who have dyslexia may have a predisposition to inattention. When such children have difficulties reading and writing, they lose interest in their studies, and their mind wanders. It is important not to miss these diagnoses. There are comorbid conditions like autism spectrum disorder that one should be aware of. To add to the complexity, dyslexia can be present as a comorbidity with ADHD.

Epidemiology[8,9]

Some 3 to 10 per cent of the population have ADHD, making it one of the commonest neurodevelopmental disorders in the world. Because the diagnosis of ADHD is imprecise, the epidemiology can be quite variable.

The ratio of males to females is just over 2:1.[10] The question is whether or not there are fewer girls with ADHD because recent studies have confirmed that girls are often underdiagnosed.

Comparison of the epidemiology of ADHD in different countries is inconsistent. Overall, there does not seem to be a significant difference between the prevalence of ADHD in Asian, African, American or European countries.[11] However, personal communications from many preschool and primary school teachers and principals have indicated that non-Asians tend to be more active in an Asian classroom.

Components of ADHD

Before we explore the causes of ADHD, we need to define some of the components of ADHD that will crop up during our discussions:

(a) **What is attention?**
   This is the ability to concentrate and maintain one's focus. Looking at it from another point of view, it is the ability to filter out extraneous noise. Young children are more susceptible to inattention, and after a few years, they can fix their attention quite well.

(b) **What is working memory?**
Most people regard working memory synonymous with short-term memory, but there is some debate about this. This is the ability to store an average of seven numbers, letters or words for 20–30 seconds. Recent studies have shown that working memory is stored in the prefrontal and parietal cortex.

(c) **What is executive function?**
Executive function is a higher order of cognitive control that enables us to reason, to solve problems, organise, prioritise, and plan complex tasks. It involves the prefrontal cortex. But when we become unable to take control of our activities or to prioritise our tasks, we lose our executive function. Most people with ADHD will have impaired executive function, but loss of executive function can occur in people who do not have ADHD. Understanding why loss of executive function may or may not be related to ADHD will help us understand the pathophysiology of ADHD.

Brain investigations

We use the following investigations to try to gain a deeper understanding into ADHD:

Brain imaging[12]

Magnetic resonance imaging and the more recent functional magnetic resonance imaging scans of the brain have helped delineate the anatomical and functional areas of the brain affected by ADHD. The following areas have shown altered functions in ADHD subjects:

(a) **Frontal cortex:** This is involved in high level functions, including attention and executive function.

(b) **Limbic System:** This regulates emotions and attention.

(c) **Basal ganglia:** Deficiency in this area can cause inter-brain communication and information to short-circuit, and contribute towards ADHD.

(d) **Reticular activating system:** This major relay system allows many pathways to enter and leave the brain; deficiency can cause inattention and hyperactivity.

Electroencephalography[13]

In some studies, the electroencephalogram of ADHD subjects showed an increase in the theta slow wave in the fronto-central electrodes. It is not present in other studies, and the findings are inconsistent. It is therefore not helpful in the diagnosis of ADHD.

Neurotransmitters[14]

Low levels of two neurotransmitters, noradrenaline and dopamine, have been found in some areas of the brain. Lack of these neurotransmitters can decrease conduction of neurons, and understanding the mechanism can help explain the drug treatment of ADHD.

Causes of ADHD[15]

Genetics[16,17]

Identical twin studies indicate that the hereditability of the disorder ranges between 60 to 80 per cent. In non-identical twins, the likelihood of the other twin getting ADHD is 50 per cent. The chances of a younger or older sibling also having the same diagnosis is 30 per cent, which compares with a 3 to 10 per cent risk in the general population.

To date, there are no predominant gene mutations thought to cause ADHD, although large numbers of gene variations have been discovered to be associated with ADHD. Some are quite interesting, especially those that are involved in dopamine neurotransmission. Another interesting finding is that there seems to be an equal distribution of the gene mutations between males and females.

Environmental factors

There is a correlation between the following risk factors and ADHD. Although correlation does not necessarily mean causation, there is a high index of suspicion that these factors could be responsible, at least in part, for provoking ADHD.

- **Maternally related prenatal risks**
  Alcohol consumption during pregnancy
  Smoking during pregnancy
  Drug use in pregnancy
  Maternal stress in pregnancy
  Maternal health in pregnancy (e.g. obesity)
- **Pregnancy and birth complications**
  Uterine-placental bleeding in pregnancy
  Protracted labour or complicated delivery
  Prematurity or low birth weight or intrauterine poor growth
  Low Apgar score at birth
- **External agents**
  Maternal-foetal Infections e.g. rubella, CMV, toxoplasmosis, etc.
  Exposure to lead and other toxins e.g., polychlorinated biphenyls
  Nutritional deficiencies
  Psychosocial effects on mother

Currently we believe there are multiple causes of ADHD and the above risk factors probably overlap with each other. Research is ongoing.

Treatment[18]

For mild ADHD and for parents who refuse medication, the recommended management of ADHD is behavioural therapy.

For more severe cases, there are several types of medicine available. A popular medicine used is methylphenidate.

Methylphenidate is a stimulant drug that blocks the reuptake of dopamine and noradrenaline by neurons. The short-acting version (Ritalin) is given orally and its effects are noticeable within half an hour, and the effects last from four to six hours. The long-acting slow-release medicine (Concerta) starts acting after one hour and it lasts from eight to 12 hours. Side effects include loss of appetite, loss of sleep, anxiety, and nausea. When given with food, or taken after food, the appetite is not affected. When given in the daytime and not giving it before sleep, there is no loss of sleep.

If teachers are not informed that their student is taking methylphenidate, they often volunteer an opinion to the parents saying that their child's behaviour has transformed for the better. The student is better behaved, less hyperactive, more focused in their studies, and the exam results show significant improvement.

If a child is unable to take methylphenidate, the alternative is atomoxetine (Strattera). This blocks the nerves from reuptaking the neurotransmitter noradrenaline. This medicine is better tolerated than methylphenidate, but it is less effective. Most of the side effects are gastrointestinal, including nausea, vomiting, heartburn, loss of appetite, and weight loss.

The other stimulant medication used for ADHD is dextroamphetamine. A double-blind crossover trial showed that both methylphenidate and dextroamphetamine were effective, but neither showed any advantage over the other.[19]

As a child gets older, and the hyperactivity becomes less prominent, some are able to stop medication. However, ADHD is a lifelong condition, and many continue taking medicine for a very long time.

Neurofeedback therapy[20]

Neurofeedback is a form of biofeedback therapy that uses real-time brain activity recorded by electroencephalogram (EEG) obtained from electrical recording leads placed on the ADHD person's scalp. Typically neurofeedback is presented by video displays or using sounds. Using operant conditioning, the person is trained to modify their brainwave patterns. Employing a system of rewards to encourage preferred brain activities, one can help the individual reduce inattention and hyperactive behaviour. Neurofeedback therapy is still not mainstream, and there is still some doubt as to whether it is effective.

Famous people with ADHD[21,22]

Creativity is the hallmark of many famous people whom we think may have ADHD. It is postulated that when your mind is overactive, you tend to think of a wider range of topics, and when you link disparate ideas together, you might stumble upon something truly original.

Richard Branson, founder of the Virgin Group, is a self-confessed ADHD, although he has not been officially diagnosed. Emma Watson who became famous when she acted in the Harry Potter movies, took medicine for ADHD.

Conclusions[23]

ADHD is one of the most fascinating diseases because there are so many unknowns and unexplored paths. The diagnosis is nebulous, and the causes are largely undetermined. How medicine exert its actions is controversial. How are so many people with ADHD not handicapped by the condition, and go on to achieve so much in their lives? For the curious-minded, ADHD is an ocean worth exploring for the hidden treasures hidden deep within.

References

1. Soreff S. Attention deficit hyperactivity disorder. Medscape 2021. https://emedicine.medscape.com/article/289350-overview#showall

2. Wikipedia. Attention deficit hyperactivity disorder. https://en.wikipedia.org/wiki/Attention_deficit_hyperactivity_disorder

3. Centers for Disease Control and Prevention. American Psychiatric Association Diagnostic and Statistical Manual 5th edition (DSM-V) test for ADHD. Centers for Disease Control and Prevention 2021. https://www.cdc.gov/ncbddd/adhd/diagnosis.html

4. Bhandari S. ADHD tests. WebMD 2022. https://www.webmd.com/add-adhd/childhood-adhd/adhd-tests-making-assessment

5. The TOVA Company. The Test of Variables of Attention (TOVA). The TOVA Company 2021 https://www.tovatest.com/

6. National Institute for Children's Health Quality. Vanderbilt assessment scales. National Institute for Children's Health Quality 2002. https://www.nichq.org/resource/nichq-vanderbilt-assessment-scales

7. Belanger SA et al. ADHD in children and youth. Paediatrics & Child Health 2018; 23: 447–453. https://www.ncbi.nlm.nih.gov/pmc/articles/PMC6199644/

8. CHADD. General prevalence of ADHD. CHADD. https://chadd.org/about-adhd/general-prevalence/

9. Psychology Today. What is ADHD (and its prevalence). https://www.psychologytoday.com/sg/basics/adhd

10. Ramdekkar UP et al. Sex and age differences in attention-deficit/hyperactivity disorder symptoms and diagnoses. Journal of the American Academy of Child and Adolescent Psychiatry 2010. https://www.ncbi.nlm.nih.gov/pmc/articles/PMC3101894/

11. Liu A et al. The prevalence of attention deficit/hyperactivity disorder among Chinese children and adolescents. Scientific Reports 2018. https://www.nature.com/articles/s41598-018-29488-2

12. Paloyelis Y et al. Functional magnetic resonance imaging in attention deficit hyperactivity disorder (ADHD). Expert Review of Neurotherapeutics 2014. https://www.ncbi.nlm.nih.gov/pmc/articles/PMC3763932/

13. Lenartowitz K & Loo SK. Use of EEG to diagnose ADHD. Current Psychiatry Reports 2014. https://www.ncbi.nlm.nih.gov/pmc/articles/PMC4633088/

14. Silver L. ADHD Neuroscience 101. ADDitude 2021. https://www.additudemag.com/adhd-neuroscience-101/

15. Thapar A et al. What causes attention deficit hyperactivity disorder? Archives of Disease in Childhood 2012; 97: 260–265. https://www.ncbi.nlm.nih.gov/pmc/articles/PMC3927422/

16. Nichols H. Is ADHD genetic? Medical News Today 2019. https://www.medicalnewstoday.com/articles/325594#is-adhd-genetic

17. Thapar A. Discoveries on the genetics of ADHD in the 21st century. Psychiatry 2018. https://ajp.psychiatryonline.org/doi/10.1176/appi.ajp.2018.18040383

18. British National Health Service (NHS). Treatment attention deficit hyperactivity disorder. NHS 2021. https://www.nhs.uk/conditions/attention-deficit-hyperactivity-disorder-adhd/treatment/

19. Efron D et al. Methylphenidate vs dexamphetamine in children with ADHD. Pediatrics 1997. https://doi.org/10.1542/peds.100.6.e6

20. Enriquez-Geppert S et al. Neurofeedback as a treatment intervention in ADHD. Current Psychiatry Reports 2019; 21: 46. https://www.ncbi.nlm.nih.gov/pmc/articles/PMC6538574/

21. Goodman DW. Famous people with ADHD. Adult Attention Deficit Disorder Center of Maryland. https://addadult.com/add-education-center/famous-people-with-adhd/

22. Montijo S. 33 famous faces of ADHD. Greatist 2019. https://greatist.com/health/adhd-celebrities#historical-figures-with-adhd

23. MentalHealthLiteracy.org. Teen Mental Health Speaks. ADHD (download). MentalHealthLiteracy.org. https://mentalhealthliteracy.org/product/tmh-speaks-adhd/

16 Dyslexia

Introduction

"He cannot read simple words like 'dog' or 'car'," the mother told me. Unable to read simple words, this six-and-a-half--year-old boy, like many others, was labelled by his teachers and classmates as lazy, dumb, or stupid. Even his parents missed the diagnosis of dyslexia because they thought that he had attention deficit hyperactivity disorder, and therefore could not concentrate on learning to read. I confirmed that he could not read, and he even wrote his own name wrongly. He was otherwise quite intelligent.

Definition[1]

The International Dyslexia Association defines dyslexia as a condition marked by difficulties with accurate and/or fluent word recognition and by poor spelling and decoding abilities. It is the commonest neurodevelopmental disorder.

Dyslexia is a lifelong condition but with intervention, the problems of understanding and working with language can be significantly reduced. Because reading and writing form a major component of our education system, children who are slow in these abilities are often labelled as "learning disabled". Dyslexics often jumble up their letters and have difficulty associating a sound with a letter, such that even familiar words are difficult to read. There is quite a wide spectrum of dyslexia, ranging from mild to severe difficulties in reading, listening to words, spelling and writing. Dyslexia is not linked to intelligence, but difficulty reading instructions can affect the intelligence test score.

Developmental language disorder (DLD) (diagnostic and statistical manual 5th edition DSM-V)[2,3]

There is another condition with symptoms that overlaps with dyslexia, but is now considered a separate entity. Known as Developmental Language Disorder (DLD), these children have no, or hardly any problems recognising words, but they cannot understand their meaning. DLD was previously known as Specific Language Impairment. Originally, it was thought that DLD was part of dyslexia, but a less severe form, appearing in slightly older children.

The difference between these two conditions is that the main problem of dyslexics is their inability to decipher the sounds of words and connect them with the visual written words. In contrast, people with DLD can hear and see the words but cannot interpret what they mean. Thus, they are thought to have problems with semantics (the meaning of words), syntax (the arrangements of words and phrases), and discourse (the formal orderly expression of thoughts delivered through speech or writing). DLD is therefore considered to be a higher level of processing deficit.

Epidemiology

The prevalence of dyslexia ranges from 7 to 15 per cent, with an average of about 10 per cent, while the prevalence of DLD is slightly lower at, or below, 7 per cent.[4] Dyslexia is the commonest learning problem.

Epidemiological studies[5] show a male predominance ranging from 1.5:1 to 3.3:1. There have been some comments that perhaps females are underdiagnosed because they are less frequently referred to diagnosticians. The reason why males are more frequently finger-pointed and referred, is because dyslexic males tend to have more unruly behaviour and express their frustrations more physically in class. This male-female inequality is still being studied and debated.

Early diagnosis[6]

It is unusual to diagnose dyslexia under the age of one year. Most children are diagnosed after the age of two years. One only suspects the diagnosis when a child learns new words very slowly, or takes much longer learning to form sentences, finds rhyming challenging, is unable to distinguish between different word sounds, reverses sounds in words, or confuses words that sound alike. At nursery school or kindergarten, they may display difficulty with spelling, avoid activities that involve reading, spend a long time trying to complete reading or writing-related tasks, read below the level expected of their age, have difficulty copying from a book or board, have difficulty remembering or understanding what they hear, are unable to pronounce unfamiliar words, or have difficulty finding words to express their thoughts.

The British Dyslexia Association lists the following early signs that should raise your suspicion of the diagnosis of dyslexia.[7]

- Finds it hard to learn nursery rhymes, has difficulty learning to sing or recite the alphabet
- Likes listening to stories but shows no interest in letters or words
- Poor auditory discrimination and can muddle up words e.g. "cubumber", "flutterby"
- Substitutes words e.g. "lampshade" for "lamppost"
- Difficulty keeping simple rhythm
- Forgets names of friends, teacher, colours, etc.
- Confuses directional words e.g. "up" and "down"
- Finds it hard to carry out two or more instructions at one time, (e.g. "put the toys inside the box, then put it on the shelf") but is fine if tasks are presented in smaller units
- Difficulty with sequencing e.g. threading a specific sequence of coloured beads, carrying out classroom routines
- Appears not to be listening or paying attention
- Unable to sit still in class
- Has a history of slow speech development
- Obvious 'good' and 'bad' days for no apparent reason
- Trouble with writing, illegible or variable handwriting
- Family history of dyslexia or reading difficulties

Genetic causes[8,9]

Dyslexia often runs in families, suggesting that there is a genetic component, and indeed, this is considered the commonest cause. Some people develop dyslexia after a brain injury arising from an infection, trauma, or a stroke, and fortunately, these "environmental" causes are relatively rare.

The genetic mutations related to dyslexia include a deletion of the DCDC2 gene which is associated with the eyes detecting fine visual movements.[10] Another mutation found in dyslexic individuals involves the ROBO1 gene, which links the auditory pathway to other parts of the brain.[11] These, and many more gene mutations, are believed to converge to cause dyslexia.

Studying genes is important as they control protein synthesis and neural connections, among their many functions. Hence, research into this area can provide further insights into the pathophysiology of dyslexia.

Brain imaging studies[12,13]

Functional magnetic resonance imaging (fMRI) scans the whole brain and shows the connectivity between different regions. Weaker connections in certain parts of the brain correlate with dyslexia. Brain imaging studies have shown that there are differences in how the dyslexic brain is structured and how it functions.

Controversy: Phonological Deficit Hypothesis[14]

Is dyslexia a problem of hearing, reading, or understanding language? In other words, is it an auditory problem, a visual problem, or a problem of making sense of words? One of the earlier theories of dyslexia is the Phonological Deficit Hypothesis.

The basis of this hypothesis is founded on the observation that reading is a complicated process and starts with recognising individual words and sounds. Each word can be dissected into smaller sound elements which are known as phonemes. For example, the word "cat" can be broken down into three phonemes: "kuh", "aah", and "tuh". Dyslexics have problems segregating the words into distinct phonemic elements. This makes it difficult for them to match specific sounds to specific letters. For example, they may have difficulty distinguishing "volcano" from "tornado". This inability to join sounds to letters is the basis of the Phonological Deficit Hypothesis.

However, this hypothesis has been challenged, and it has currently fallen out of favour. Nevertheless, it forms the basis of a therapy popularly used in the management of dyslexia, called the Orton-Gillingham Approach.[15] This technique helps break words down into their component sounds, match the sounds to the letters, and then blend these sounds together. This therapy employs a multisensory approach. For example, children might be asked to trace letters in sand, or clap out syllables when reciting words. There is no convincing evidence to date that this technique improves dyslexia.

Problems associated with dyslexia[16]

Children who have dyslexia have difficulty reading and writing, and take a longer time to understand what they are taught. They tend to do poorly in spelling tests and school exams, which will lower their self-esteem, and some may even become anxious and depressed. They are also at increased risk of having impulsive behaviours and attention deficit hyperactivity disorder.

The Mayo Clinic lists the following problems if someone with dyslexia is untreated:

- Learning difficulties: Because reading and writing are basic skills for most school subjects, a child with dyslexia is at a disadvantage and may have trouble keeping up with their peers.
- Social problems: Left untreated, dyslexic children may have low self-esteem, behavioural problems, anxiety, aggression, and exhibit withdrawal from friends, parents and teachers.
- Problems in later life: The inability to read and comprehend can prevent a child from reaching his or her potential as the child grows up. This can have long-term educational, social and economic consequences.

Tips for parents on how to manage dyslexia

1. Start reading to your child from a young age. Interest them with picture books and use emotions to represent the different characters in the story. Point to words of interest in the book. Get your child to guess what happens next in the story. Make reading an enjoyable positive experience.

2. In an older child, get them to read back parts of the story to you, gently giving corrective feedback. You can also monitor how long it takes for your child to read a short passage. Children can enjoy being timed, and they take delight in seeing if they can improve their speed. Repeating the reading of a passage can improve fluency.

3. Build vocabulary. Ask your child to inform you of the new words they have learnt every day. Talk about the words, their meaning(s), placing the words in sentences, and checking on their meaning in a dictionary. Play word games where you try to insert new words into a sentence; do it at least twice that day, then again later that week. Write down the daily list of new words and run through them weekly.

4. Play games. Engage your child by playing fun word games. For example, clap with each syllable of a word spoken out loud. Separate the components of a multisyllabic word, and join them back together. Point out alliterations (sound duplications) in songs, poems, and nursery rhymes.

5. Go high-tech. Do not be afraid to use computer resources, apps, and digital learning games. Instruction must be explicit, motivating, systematic, and supportive. Be guided by what the teacher is also teaching in the classroom. But do not spend too much time on the computer at home in case your child becomes too addicted to it.

Practical classroom management

(a) Students learn more effectively in small groups (less than six children per teacher) but this may not always be achievable in some schools. Ideally, the teachers should have received training in teaching children how to read.

(b) Try introducing and talking around the subject matter before reading the text. Whenever possible, relate the text to real life experiences. Enhance the teaching with pictures, common household items, outdoor activities and field trips.

(c) Increase vocabulary by selecting practical high-utility words, e.g. "living", "order", "ground", "course". Apply the new words in conversation and in writing. Teach proper pronunciation by reading the words correctly, e.g. "there", "strike", "grasp". Learn how words are derived from root segments, and join them up into different words;

for example take these root fragments: "auto", "vac", and join them up into words like "automobile", "vacate". Alternatively, you can split a long word into their components, like: "triangle", "loveable". If the word has several meanings when used in different contexts, talk about them (e.g. "bat", "lead"). Explore figures of speech, synonyms and homophones, and try to give concrete applications of these words (e.g. "heart of stone", "raining cats and dogs").

(d) Teach the rules of language, correct spelling and the exceptions where the rules are allowed to be broken. For example, different spelling of words that sound alike: "hair" and "hare".

(e) Get the child to read texts pitched at their level. Use the same words in different contexts, and try fluency drills with repeat practice using the same words. For example, "jam" used as a noun is different from its use as a verb.

Bilingualism[17] (also see Chapter 9)

Some teachers and colleagues advise parents and caregivers of dyslexic children to avoid bilingual language use at home. Research evidence does not show any advantages or disadvantages of dyslexics speaking more than one language. Certainly, bilingualism is not a cause of dyslexia. Converting into monolingual conversations at home also shows no advantages. Some have suggested that bilingualism might even benefit dyslexics learning to read, but there is no evidence to support this claim either.[17]

Different languages and different countries[18,19]

What is fascinating is the comparison of the prevalence of dyslexia in different countries. One study showed that the prevalence of dyslexia in China is 3.9 per cent,[20] which is lower than that of several Western countries, which ranges from 5 to 17 per cent. But before you draw the conclusion that pictographic languages like Chinese are less likely to result in dyslexia, studies of Japanese dyslexics came to the opposite conclusion. The difference between dyslexics in hiragana, the Japanese alphabet is very low, at 1 per cent. In contrast, the prevalence of dyslexics using the kanji pictogram is higher at 5 to 6 per cent.

Researching the mechanisms of language learning is important in getting into the fundamental understanding of brain function. How different languages can affect behaviour and personalities is another interesting area of research.

New technology[21]

There are many new ways to help dyslexics, and the number of new devices and programmes is increasing. Here are some that are currently available.

1. Dragon Naturally Speaking transcribes spoken into written words, and translates the words into other languages.
2. Natural Reader is the opposite of Dragon Naturally Speaking, in that it converts the written text into speech. It also has an inbuilt translator so that the speech can be delivered in another language.
3. Livescribe Smart Pen facilitates writing on a computer, and has other functions including audio recording.
4. New fonts with letters designed to be heavier at the bottom, so as to prevent readers turning the letters upside down.
5. fMRI can observe in real time the areas of the brain used in speech and reading. This enables one to diagnose dyslexia, as well as to assess which therapy is most effective in training the dyslexic brain to speak, read and write.

History of dyslexia[22]

From an evolutionary viewpoint, humans differ from other animals in their ability to communicate using a more sophisticated language. It started with spoken words. Then about 5,500 years ago in Mesopotamia, written cuneiform language appeared. In terms of the evolutionary time scale, written language is quite a recent development, and therefore did not have the millions of years required to embed the survival advantage into our genes.

Doctors and medical students might remember the name Adolph Kussmaul, who described the slow sighing breathing found in some diabetics, and which is now known as Kussmaul respiration. In 1877, he coined the term "word-blindness" to describe patients who had difficulty reading. Ten years later, in 1887, German ophthalmologist Rudolf Berlin first used the term "dyslexia" to describe the patients who despite having good eyesight, were unable to read written words. In 1896, the British physician William Pringle Morgan first identified the condition in a child, and described the symptoms of dyslexia in greater detail.

Famous dyslexics[23]

The list of famous dyslexics is very long. We suspect, but cannot prove, whether those famous people who are no longer with us, really did have dyslexia. Take Leonardo da Vinci, for example, of whom we have reason to think had dyslexia. He drew and wrote with his left hand, and was able to write mirror image effortlessly (a feature of many dyslexics), and frequently made spelling mistakes, especially in homophonic words.

It is also interesting to note that 35 per cent of entrepreneurs are dyslexic, compared to 10 per cent of the general population. These dyslexic entrepreneurs appear to be good at creating new ideas; they are also often good at speaking and delegating tasks.

The question all of us are asking is why so many world-famous brilliant people are dyslexic. One would have thought that the inability to read and write fluently must be a handicap. So why have so many of them accomplished such incredible achievements, and been labelled geniuses?

One popular theory is that if you are handicapped in one area, you will overcome the difficulty by compensating for it and excelling in another area. For example, the blind can hear sounds more sharply, and touch objects more sensitively, while the deaf can see more clearly. What seems quite counter-intuitive are the famous writers who confess that they suffer from dyslexia; examples include F Scott Fitzgerald, William Butler Yeats, Hans Christian Andersen, and Agatha Christie. We must not forget one famous lawyer who became Singapore's prime minister and who was dyslexic, Lee Kuan Yew.

Conclusions[24–26]

Dyslexia is a common condition affecting around 10 per cent of the general population. Early recognition can help the affected persons become more fluent in reading, writing and understanding language. This will have psychological and other benefits like increasing academic performance and self-confidence. Research into the mechanisms of dyslexia, and the different forms it takes in different languages, and the influence of different cultures, can help deepen one's understanding of how we acquire knowledge and communicate with one another. Hopefully, we will gain insights into our thinking processes, personality, creativity and our ultimate success.

References

1. International Dyslexia Association, Inc. Definition of dyslexia. International Dyslexia Association, Inc. https://dyslexiaida.org/definition-of-dyslexia/

2. Catts HW *et al.* Are specific language impairment and dyslexia distinct disorders? Journal of Speech, Language, and Hearing Research 2005; 48: 1378–1396. https://www.ncbi.nlm.nih.gov/pmc/articles/PMC2853030/

3. Snowling M. Dyslexia and developmental language disorder: same or different? Association for Child and Adolescent Mental Health 2017. https://www.acamh.org/blog/dyslexia-developmental-language-disorder-different/

4. Laasonen M *et al.* Understanding developmental language disorder. BMC Psychology 2018; 6: 24. https://www.ncbi.nlm.nih.gov/pmc/articles/PMC5963016/

5. Arnett AB *et al.* Explaining the sex difference in dyslexia. The Journal of Child Psychology and Psychiatry 2017; 58: 719–727. https://www.ncbi.nlm.nih.gov/pmc/articles/PMC5438271/

6. The Yale Center for Dyslexia & Creativity. Suspect dyslexia? Act early. The Yale Center for Dyslexia & Creativity. https://dyslexia.yale.edu/resources/parents/what-parents-can-do/suspect-dyslexia-act-early/

7. The British Dyslexia Association. Is my child dyslexic? Signs of dyslexia, early years. The British Dyslexia Association. https://www.bdadyslexia.org.uk/advice/children/is-my-child-dyslexic/signs-of-dyslexia-early-years

8. Hensler BS *et al.* Behavioral genetic approach to the study of dyslexia. Journal of Developmental & Behavioral Pediatrics 2010; 31: 525–532. https://www.ncbi.nlm.nih.gov/pmc/articles/PMC2952936/

9. Schumacher J *et al.* Genetics of dyslexia: the evolving landscape. Journal of Medical Genetics 2007; 44: 289–297. https://www.ncbi.nlm.nih.gov/pmc/articles/PMC2597981/

10. Chen Y *et al.* DCDC2 gene polymorphisms are associated with developmental dyslexia in Chinese Uyghur children. Neural Regeneration Research 2017; 12: 259–266. https://www.ncbi.nlm.nih.gov/pmc/articles/PMC5361510/

11. Hannula-Jouppi K *et al*. The axon guidance receptor gene ROBO1 is a candidate gene for developmental dyslexia. PLoS Genetics 2005; 1: e50. https://www.ncbi.nlm.nih.gov/pmc/articles/PMC1270007/

12. The International Dyslexia Association. Dyslexia and the brain. The International Dyslexia Association. https://dyslexiaida.org/dyslexia-and-the-brain-fact-sheet/

13. Elnakib A *et al*. Magnetic resonance imaging findings for dyslexia. Journal of Biomedical Nanotechnology 2014; 10: 2778–2805. https://www.researchgate.net/publication/269993420_Magnetic_Resonance_Imaging_Findings_for_Dyslexia_A_Review

14. Wikipedia. Phonological deficit hypothesis https://en.wikipedia.org/wiki/Phonological_deficit_hypothesis

15. Wikipedia. Orton-Gillingham. https://en.wikipedia.org/wiki/Orton-Gillingham

16. Mayo Clinic Staff. Dyslexia. Mayo Clinic 2017. https://www.mayoclinic.org/diseases-conditions/dyslexia/symptoms-causes/syc-20353552#

17. Rosen P. FAQs about bilingualism and dyslexia. Understood for All Inc. https://www.understood.org/en/learning-thinking-differences/child-learning-disabilities/dyslexia/faqs-about-bilingualism-and-dyslexia

18. Husni H & Jamaluddin Z. A retrospective and future look at speech recognition applications in assisting children with reading disabilities. http://www.iaeng.org/publication/WCECS2008/WCECS2008_pp555-558.pdf https://www.researchgate.net/publication/44262361_A_Retrospective_and_Future_Look_at_Speech_Recognition_Applications_in_Assisting_Children_with_Reading_Disabilities

19. Butterworth B & Tang J. Dyslexia has a language barrier. The Guardian 2004. https://www.theguardian.com/education/2004/sep/23/research.highereducation2

20. Sun Z *et al*. Prevalence and associated risk factors of dyslexic children in a middle-sized city of China. PLOS ONE 2013. https://journals.plos.org/plosone/article?id=10.1371/journal.pone.0056688

21. Nixon G. How technology Is changing treatments for dyslexia. Gemm Learning 2015. https://www.gemmlearning.com/blog/dyslexia/technology-is-changing-treatments-for-dyslexia/

22. The British Psychological Society. The history of dyslexia. Oxford Psychologist. https://dyslexiahistory.web.ox.ac.uk/brief-history-dyslexia

23. Davis Dyslexia Association International. List of dyslexic achievers. Davis Dyslexia Association International. https://www.dyslexia.com/about-dyslexia/dyslexic-achievers/all-achievers/

24. Marianne. Free dyslexia resources. Homeschooling with Dyslexia 2017. https://homeschoolingwithdyslexia.com/free-dyslexia-resources/

25. Elbeheri G, Siang L. The Routledge International Handbook of Dyslexia in Education. Routledge 2022. ISBN 9780367754488
26. Snowling MJ. Dyslexia: A very short introduction. Oxford University Press 2019. ISBN 9780198818304

Online help

Dyslexia Association of Singapore (DAS)
Telephone (+65) 6444 5700
Email: info@das.org.sg
Website: https://www.das.org.sg/

17 Depression and suicide

Rise in suicides[1,2]

Today I learnt that one of my students' close friend had committed suicide. And only a few months ago, one of my colleagues' son had also committed suicide. It is devastating for these families when their young ones, in their early 20s, end their lives.

Newspapers have reported a surge in suicides especially during the COVID-19 pandemic. Why do people take their own lives? How does the COVID-19 pandemic contribute to the rise in depression and suicides? This will be discussed later. But first, let us define depression.

What is depression?[3-5]

It is a feeling of sadness that is felt more intensely and lasts longer than the transient heartaches, disappointments and blues that we all encounter in our daily lives.

Clinical presentation

There's a difference between "having depression" and "feeling sad". We all feel very despondent when we fail an exam, get rejected by an institution of tertiary education, or lose our job. We feel sad, but after a while, we pull ourselves together and overcome this temporary unhappiness. In contrast, clinical depression lingers on for much longer, sometimes for two weeks or more. It interferes significantly with our studying, working, playing, eating and sleeping.

Symptoms of depression[6]

The following symptoms are listed in the American Psychiatric Association's Diagnostic and Statistical Manual 5th Edition (DSM-5):

- Low mood, feeling sad most of the day, occurring nearly every day
- Loss of interest in things one normally enjoys
- Changes in appetite leading to significant weight loss or gain
- Feeling restless, agitated, pacing up and down, psychomotor impairment like slowing of thoughts and movements
- Extreme fatigue, loss of energy
- Feeling of worthlessness or excessive guilt
- Poor concentration, lowered ability to think or pay attention
- Inability to sleep, or oversleeping
- Recurrent thoughts of suicide or have attempted suicide

Diagnosis[7]

According to the DSM-5, you need five or more of the above symptoms to qualify for a diagnosis of depression, On top of that, there are the following additional requirements: These symptoms must cause significant distress to one's daily life. They cannot be due to the consumption of medicine known to be associated with depression. One needs to exclude substance abuse, and other medical or mental conditions, such as a schizoaffective disorder. There cannot be a manic or hypomanic episode at any point.

Depression can affect males and females all the way from early childhood to old age. No socioeconomic status or ethnic groups are exempt from depression.

Other symptoms associated with depression

We have listed above the official DSM-5 symptoms of depression, but most people who have been working with individuals who suffer from this condition are aware of other symptoms listed below, and these should be looked out for as well:

- Irritability and anger
- Memory loss

- Self-blame
- Brooding and rumination
- Social withdrawal
- Blunted circadian rhythm where the timing of the sleep-wake cycle is disturbed

How depression affects one's daily life

There are many ways in which depression can affect one's daily life. These include:

- Hampering academic studies or work performance
- Disrupting meaningful relationships with others
- Slowing down in getting things done
- Eating a poor diet and becoming malnourished

Depression in children[8–11]

Depression in children is quite difficult to pick up, and the diagnosis is often delayed or missed. Symptoms may not be constant, and can fluctuate from day to day, depending on the environment and events. As a child grows up, the manifestations of depression can unfold differently at different ages. One must have a high index of suspicion if a child has continuous feelings of sadness or hopelessness, if there are bouts of anger or crankiness, or if they become socially withdrawn, display changes in appetite or food preferences, change their sleep patterns, have difficulty concentrating on schoolwork, cry a lot, or have thoughts of suicide. Some may even present with superficially unrelated symptoms like headaches and abdominal pain, so caregivers and doctors should be alert to the possibility of an underlying depression.

Subtypes of depression

(a) Peripartum Depression[12]

Postpartum depression or "baby blues" usually occurs after childbirth, but studies have shown that some mothers may have depression prior to childbirth. Thus, the condition has been renamed "depressive disorder with peripartum onset". It can occur during pregnancy or up to four weeks after birth. Some 10 to 15 per cent of mothers experience postpartum depression. Symptoms include mood swings, frequent crying, trouble bonding with the baby, tiredness, fearing that they will not be a good mother, or a sense of worthlessness or shame. In women, several hormones including oestrogen, progesterone, prolactin and cortisol all decrease significantly after childbirth, and this drop may be responsible for causing the depression. Lifestyle changes may also play a role, because men can also experience depression around the same time. In men, their levels of testosterone and vasopressin fluctuate during and immediately after their female partner's pregnancy, but the precise mechanism of depression in males is still unclear. Both males and females will experience environmental changes such as dealing with an inconsolable baby, sleep deprivation, changes in one's daily routines, and having difficulty finding adequate support to take care of baby.

(b) **Atypical Depression**[13]

Atypical depression is characterised by increased sensitivity and reactions to changes in the environment. There may be improved mood during positive events, and this is referred to as "mood reactivity". This contrasts with "melancholic depression" where even previously pleasurable events do not elevate one's moods. People suffering from atypical depression may exhibit increased appetite, weight gain, heavy feeling in the limbs (leaden paralysis), oversleeping, and become extremely anxious when being scolded or rejected.

(c) **Persistent Depressive Disorder (Dysthymia)[14]**

This subtype is a chronic form of depression which lasts over a longer period of time, usually more than two years. The severity can also fluctuate over time. Symptoms include changes in appetite and sleep patterns, fatigue or low energy, reduced self-esteem and concentration, struggling to make decisions, feeling hopeless, and harbouring pessimistic thoughts.

Differential diagnosis

Bipolar disorder[15]

Bipolar disorder was formerly known as manic depression and is characterised by extreme mood swings between hyperexcitable behaviour followed by depression. Some patients are misdiagnosed as suffering from depression. One should try to find out if the person has up-and-down mood swings and manic episodes; if so, this points towards a diagnosis of bipolar disorder. The reason why it is important to make a correct diagnosis is that the treatment differs from depression. Lithium carbonate is the preferred treatment for bipolar disorder.

Seasonal affective disorder[16]

Depression that occurs either in the winter months or during spring-summer months are diagnosed as Seasonal Affective Disorder. Countries where the winter months are cold and the sun sets early resulting in dark afternoons and evenings can make some people feel rather moody and sad. It has recently been realised that there is also depression that can occur during the spring and summer months. It is thought that this form of depression is due to allergy to pollen.

Causes[17–19]

The causes of depression are still not fully worked out. A lot of research has been conducted utilising advanced technology, and the results are still coming in.

Genetics[20]

If a first-degree relative has depression, then one has a higher risk of getting depression too. If an identical twin has depression, the other twin has a 60 to 80 percent chance of developing it. A non-identical twin, on the other hand only has a 20 per cent chance of experiencing depression.

The vast majority of individuals suffering from depression do not have close relatives with this condition. Depression is a heterogeneous condition which often overlaps with other personality, behavioural and psychiatric disorders, and there are no laboratory or imaging techniques to make a definitive diagnosis. Is depression a single disease, or is it made up of several diseases with some common and overlapping symptoms? Without a clear-cut diagnosis critics have raised issues with current aetiology studies.

Unlike other major psychiatric disorders like autism, genetic studies of depression have not achieved promising results. Following the successful human genome project, where the entire human DNA was mapped out in 2003, several Genome Wide Associations Studies have been conducted in many countries, using large sets of samples, including thousands of patients with different forms of depression, and meta-analyses of thousands of patients scrutinised. Unfortunately, all have failed to identify any specific gene loci responsible for the predisposition to depression.

Recently, there have been some suggestions that perhaps mitochondrial dysfunction may play a role in the development of major depressive disorders. If true, this throws a spanner in the works.

Environmental factors

Life events

Tragic events, like the death of a family member, failing an exam, losing a job, getting divorced, or being bullied, can increase the chances of having depression. A traumatic childhood, sexual or psychological abuse, neglect, poverty, and unhealthy lifestyles, can also predispose one to develop depression later in life. The side effects of certain medicines, like corticosteroids, beta-blockers, and statins (treatment of high cholesterol levels), can result in depression. Recreational drugs, like amphetamines, can also lead to depression.

Based on a combination of genetic and environmental factors, it is postulated that depression has neurochemical and neurostructural aetiologies.

Neuropathology of depression[21,22]

The commonest theory about the cause of depression is the theory of chemical imbalance in the brain, especially the lack of serotonin, the "feel good chemical". This is based on the observation that raising the level of serotonin through medicine can alleviate symptoms of depression in some patients. However, this view does not really capture the complexity of depression.

(a) Monoamine deficiency theory[23]

The monoamine deficiency theory was proposed when it was discovered that the treatment of depression elevated the levels of monoamine neurotransmitters.

These monoamine neurotransmitters include serotonin, noradrenaline and dopamine. Each of them may have an impact on separate sets of symptoms:

- Serotonin: obsessions and compulsions
- Noradrenaline: anxiety and attention
- Dopamine: attention, motivation and pleasure

Low levels of serotonin which can be induced by depleting tryptophan, the amino acid which is used to make serotonin, can lead to symptoms of depression. It also links to DNA studies of depression.

However, there are some problems with the monoamine theory. Medicines used in the treatment of depression can quickly raise monoamine levels, but improvements in symptoms lag behind by several weeks. Not everyone who was given antidepressant medicines showed improvement in their depression. Drugs that did the opposite and lowered monoamine levels did not always cause depression. Many studies showed inconsistent correlation between monoamine levels and their neurotransmission with the symptoms, so this theory is currently considered inadequate.

(b) Neural Growth and Connections Theory[24]

In recent years, scientists have discovered that brain cell growth and connections may play a larger role in the cause of depression. The hippocampus tends to be much smaller in depressed patients. The hippocampus is the area of the brain that controls memories and emotions. The longer the person has been depressed, the smaller the hippocampus becomes. Stress may be the main trigger to decrease the number of new neurons in this area of the brain. When this area of the brain regenerates and new neurons are stimulated, the mood improves. Many drugs, especially those that affect serotonin levels, have an indirect effect on the growth of brain cells. Nerve cells that secrete serotonin also secrete other chemicals that stimulate growth of new neurons or neurogenesis.

Investigations

Magnetic Resonance Imaging (MRI)[25]

Magnetic resonance imaging shows structural changes in the brain in patients with depression. The front part of the brain known as the prefrontal cortex has a portion known as the ventromedial cortex, which is much smaller in depressed individuals compared to that of normal individuals. The ventromedial cortex enables an individual to be stimulated by positive rewards and experience pleasure. It also enables one to switch from one mood to another. The cells involved in this function are the glial cells which supply nerve cells with energy, and the number of these cells is decreased in depressed patients.

Positron Emission Tomography (PET) scan and functional magnetic resonance imaging[26,27]

Positron Emission Tomography (PET) Scan allows scientists to determine the metabolic rates of the brain by measuring oxygen and blood sugar (glucose) utilisation. Findings from PET scans have been confirmed by functional MRI. The latter looks at the blood flow into different areas of the brain. Using both these techniques, scientists have discovered that depressed people have less activity in the prefrontal cortex, including the ventromedial cortex. Paradoxically, there is more blood flow to the limbic area which contains the hippocampus responsible for processing memory, despite the shrinkage of the hippocampus in depression.

Electroencephalogram (EEG)[28]

There can be changes in the rapid eye movement (REM) pattern as well as the slow wave phase of the sleep cycle. The EEG shows decreased REM sleep latency, decreased slow wave activity, and deeper delta waves in depressed subjects. This reflects the sleep disturbances reported by depressed individuals.

Blood tests

Blood is taken to exclude low thyroid hormones or hypothyroidism, high cortisol levels, vitamin deficiencies, and the presence of substance abuse drugs. Patients with high cholesterol levels may be taking statins, a potential cause of depression.

Treatments

Non-pharmacological treatments

Between 70 and 80 per cent will improve their depressive symptoms if treated correctly. Increased physical activity, going for walks, socialising more, and participation in the arts and music can all help reduce depressive symptoms.

Psychotherapy[29]

Psychotherapy, or talk therapy, can help alleviate depression, and appears to be better in maintaining long term alleviation. This includes cognitive behavioural therapy, interpersonal therapy, and psychodynamic therapy. They help the individual to focus on the present, and encourages the regaining of control over mood and function. Success for this type of therapy depends on the relationship between the patient and therapist.

Social support

Love and support from family and friends help tremendously. Strong social support leads to better long-term outcomes.

Music and art therapy[30,31]

Both music and art therapy have been shown to help people with depression. They make one feel more relaxed, soothe the mind, and lift one's spirits.

Physical activities[32]

Regular physical activities help reduce depression. Theories of why physical activity works include the increased release of neurotransmitters, and other chemicals such as endorphins and endocannabinoids which relax tense muscles. Exercising for 20 minutes three or more times per week is effective.

Diet[33]

Although the evidence linking diet and relieving depression is not absolutely definitive, it is possible that eating more fruits and vegetables may have some positive benefits.

Antidepressants

While antidepressants can alleviate depression, whether or not they will lower suicide risk is a controversial topic. Epidemiological studies have shown conflicting results, some showing increased and others showing decreased risk of suicide.[28]

(a) **Selective Serotonin Reuptake Inhibitors (SSRIs)[34]**
This group of medicines blocks the reuptake of serotonin in the brain's synaptic gap, thereby prolonging the amount of serotonin in the synapse, enhancing neurotransmission. Serotonin is associated with happiness. SSRIs are generally preferred over other types of medicine, especially in children, adolescents, and patients with late-onset depression. There are also fewer adverse reactions compared with other antidepressants. They include gastrointestinal upsets, sexual dysfunction, fatigue and restlessness.

In the 1990s, some three per cent of American were taking Prozac, an SSRI antidepressant. The prevalence of consuming antidepressants has quadrupled over the following few decades, and there used to be a joke pointing to the US as a "Prozac Nation"!

(b) **Serotonin/Noradrenaline Reupdate Inhibitors (SNRIs)[35]**
For patients who suffer from pain or extreme tiredness, the SRNIs can be considered as a first-line treatment. SRNIs should be used alone because there are some interactions when combined with other

antidepressants. Side effects include dizziness, dry mouth, diarrhoea or constipation.

(c) **Monoamine Oxidase Inhibitors**[36]

Monoamine oxidase inhibitors prevent the metabolism of the mono-amines 5-hydroxytryptamine and noradrenaline, which increases the level of these neurotransmitter monoamines. An important side effect is the risk of a hypertensive crisis. A low tyramine diet is recommended. Other side effects are insomnia, lack of sleep, anxiety, sexual dysfunction and weight gain.

(d) **Tricyclic Antidepressants (TCI)**[37]

TCIs block the reuptake of serotonin and noradrenaline in the presynaptic nerves. They were introduced in the 1950s and are currently used as a second-line treatment when other antidepressants are ineffective. They elevate one's mood. Unfortunately, side effects are more common with TCIs, and include drowsiness, blurred vision, dry mouth, constipation, urine retention. They have also been used for people with obsessive-compulsive disorder and can help some who suffer panic disorders.

(e) **N-Methyl-D-aspartate (NMDA) Antagonists**[38]

The NMDA receptor is activated by glutamate and when that happens, a nerve signal is activated. The NMDA receptor antagonist will block the receptor and hence inhibits electrical impulses from passing through. The antidepressant effects of the NMDA receptor antagonist can be felt relatively quickly, in about four hours.

ElectroConvulsive therapy[39]

A small and controlled amount of electric current is passed through the brain while the patient is under general anaesthesia. This induces a brief seizure. This procedure has been around for decades and is used for major depressive patients. It is effective in about 50 per cent of patients.

Deep brain stimulation[40]

Quite recently, neurosurgeons have reported successful treatment of several patients' severe and treatment-resistant depression by implanting a wire attached to a pacemaker-like electrical device. The wire is inserted into an area of the brain known as the subgenual cingulate region (also known as Brodmann's area 25), and a part of the middle frontal cortex. The instrument delivers continual electrical stimulation to these brain areas, with the stimulation having a pronounced antidepressant effect. Exactly why and how this treatment appears to work is unclear. Perhaps stimulation of these regions, which connects the limbic (emotion) centres in the brain with the frontal cortex allows the patient to better manage and regulate one's emotions. The frontal cortex might then help reduce depressive thoughts. Further research is in the pipeline.

Transcranial magnetic stimulation[41]

This is a non-invasive procedure using magnetic fields applied externally to stimulate part of the brain in order to alleviate depression. An electromagnetic coil delivers the magnetic waves to the frontal cortex. It is painless, safe and well-tolerated. The exact mechanism is unknown but it is speculated that the magnetic waves might stimulate that part of the brain which is underactive in people who have depression. Side effects are uncommon, and include headaches, twitching of the facial muscles, light-headedness, and some tingling sensations. It works in about 30 per cent of depressive patients and fails in 50 to 60 per cent of patients.

Suicide[42,43]

In many countries, suicide is the leading cause of death for those aged 10–29. In Singapore, over 400 lives are lost annually to suicide, which is five times more than deaths from car accidents.[1] Males account for more than 70 per cent of all suicides. The statistics show that out of seven attempted suicides, only one will succeed. We should try to prevent them all.

The risk factors

Keep a lookout for risk factors. If you hear or observe any of the following, talk to the individual, asking how things are:

- Previous attempt of taking one's life, or a family history of suicide
- Depression and other mental health problems

- Serious or chronic health conditions, terminal illness
- Distressing life events (failing exams, divorce, job loss, death of close ones, etc.)
- Prolonged stress factors (bullying, cyberbullying, physical and emotional abuse, unemployment, etc.)
- Alcoholic, substance abuse (heroin, amphetamines, etc)

The warning signs of suicidal thoughts

Listen carefully

If you hear someone say anything like the following, take what they say seriously. Do not dismiss it summarily, and do not say "Everything will be all right." Better to ask, "Is there something bothering you?" or "Are you unhappy about something?" Here are some worrying words spoken by a person who is at risk of attempting suicide:

- "My family will be better off without me"
- "My life is meaningless anyway"
- "If you don't love me, I'll kill myself"

Unusual actions or writings

If you see someone posting messages on the Internet, it is better to err on the side of caution and discuss the matter with that person. Try asking them, "Anything the matter?" or "Can we talk about what's happening?"

Writing about departing from this world, talking about sadness, and suicide notes (posting on social media, blogs, group chats, YouTube, etc.) are warning signs. Also take note of the following actions:

- Giving away treasured possessions and saying goodbye
- Researching suicide methods, buying rope

Changes in behaviour

If your son, daughter, friend or student display any of the following, you should try to help that individual:

- Emotional outbursts (anger, sadness, irritability, recklessness)
- Loss of interest in previously enjoyed activities
- Humiliation or anxiety
- Withdrawal from social activities

The COVID-19 pandemic and depression[44–46]

The COVID-19 infection rapidly spread from January 2020 engulfing the entire world and changed everyone's lives. Millions of people have caught the disease, and already millions have died from it. Jobs were lost affecting one's income, schools and restaurants restricted gatherings, theatre and music performances were curtailed. There was reduced social mobility, increased social isolation, and reduced air travel. All these factors have made people feel very lonely, resulting in heightened stress, anxiety, frustration, and hostility. It is estimated that a third of the population have shown increased anxiety and depression during the pandemic. Suicide rates have increased markedly.[1,2]

At times like this, family, friends and social organisations need to support one another. Mental health counselling services need to be increased. Governments can help by ensuring COVID-19 is under public health control, encouraging vaccinations. Economically, they can supplement lost incomes, reduce rental charges, and open up new jobs and training schemes.

Conclusions[47]

It is important to note that suicide is potentially preventable. Just talking to the depressed person can help alleviate suicidal thoughts and prevent a tragedy. Be neutral and do not be judgemental. Unfortunately, telling the person not to worry or that everything will sort itself out is probably not going to help. Better to spend time listening to the person's problems, worries, failures, suffering, and fears. Some individuals want to end their life because they want to terminate an unbearably painful situation, but if they can be shown an alternative solution, they may not embark on such an irreversible act. If you feel you are not the right person to help, look for someone else who is more likely to be effective. Sometimes you may have to talk to that person's relatives or mutual friends to make them aware of the situation. In the meantime, you can try to persuade the depressed person to talk to their relatives and friends, and seek psychological or medical or any other appropriate help.

References

1. Ang M. Overall suicide rate decreased in 2021 but increased among youths aged 10–29. Mothership 2022. https://mothership.sg/2022/07/suicide-rate-young-people-increase/

2. Choong J. On average almost four suicide cases reported to police every day, Malaysia. Malay Mail 2021. https://www.malaymail.com/news/malaysia/2021/06/29/covid-19-on-average-almost-four-suicide-cases-reported-to-police-every-day/1985906

3. Tacchi MJ & Scott J. Depression: A Very Short Introduction. Oxford University Press 2017. ISBN 9780199558650 https://global.oup.com/ukhe/product/depression-a-very-short-introduction-9780199558650?cc=gb&lang=en

4. Wikipedia. Major depressive disorder. https://en.wikipedia.org/wiki/Major_depressive_disorder

5. Halverson, JL. Depression. Medscape 2020. https://emedicine.medscape.com/article/286759-overview#showall

6. Truschel, J. Diagnostic and Statistical Manual 5th edition (DSM-V) Diagnosis of depression. Psycom 2020. https://www.psycom.net/depression-definition-dsm-5-diagnostic-criteria/

7. Smith KM et al. The diagnosis of depression: current and emerging methods. Comprehensive Psychiatry 2013; 54: 1–6. https://www.ncbi.nlm.nih.gov/pmc/articles/PMC5502713/

8. Casarella J. Depression in children. WebMD 2021. https://www.webmd.com/depression/guide/depression-children

9. Schimelpfening J. What to know about childhood depression. VeryWell Mind 2021. https://www.verywellmind.com/childhood-depression-1066805

10. Centers for Disease Control and Prevention. Anxiety and depression in children. Centers for Disease Control and Prevention 2021. https://www.cdc.gov/childrensmentalhealth/depression.html

11. Demitri M. Depression in children and adolescents. PsychCentral 2016. https://psychcentral.com/lib/depression-in-children-and-adolescents#1

12. Langan RC & Goodbred AJ. Identification and management of peripartum depression. American Family Physician 2016; 93: 852–858. https://www.aafp.org/afp/2016/0515/p852.html

13. Wikipedia. Atypical depression. https://en.wikipedia.org/wiki/Atypical_depression

14. Mayo Clinic Staff. Persistent Depressive Disorder Dysthymia. Mayo Clinic 2018. https://www.mayoclinic.org/diseases-conditions/persistent-depressive-disorder/symptoms-causes/syc-20350929

15. Mayo Clinic Staff. Bipolar disorder. Mayo Clinic 2021. https://www.mayoclinic.org/diseases-conditions/bipolar-disorder/symptoms-causes/syc-20355955

16. Mayo Clinic Staff. Seasonal Affective Disorder. Mayo Clinic 2021 https://www.mayoclinic.org/diseases-conditions/seasonal-affective-disorder/symptoms-causes/syc-20364651

17. Bruce DF. Causes of depression. WebMD 2021 https://www.webmd.com/depression/guide/causes-depression

18. MentalHelp.net. Biology of depression. MentalHelp.net. https://www.mentalhelp.net/depression/biology-genetics-and-imaging/

19. Wikipedia. Biology of depression. https://en.wikipedia.org/wiki/Biology_of_depression

20. Shadrina M et al. Genetic factors in major depression disorders. Frontiers in Psychiatry 2018. https://www.ncbi.nlm.nih.gov/pmc/articles/PMC6065213/

21. Mayberg HS et al. Reciprocal Limbic-Cortical Function and Negative Mood: Converging PET Findings in Depression and Normal Sadness. The American Journal of Psychiatry 1999. https://ajp.psychiatryonline.org/doi/full/10.1176/ajp.156.5.675

22. Kent C. MRI imaging shows physical abnormalities in depressed brain. Medical Device Network 2019. https://www.medicaldevice-network.com/news/mri-for-depression/

23. Williams S. Monoamine theory of depression exposed as incomplete, simplistic. Odyssey 2016. https://www.theodysseyonline.com/depressions-new-definition

24. Chaudhury D et al. Neuronal correlates of depression. Cellular and Molecular Life Sciences 2015; 72: 4825–4848. https://www.ncbi.nlm.nih.gov/pmc/articles/PMC4709015/

25. Kent C. MRI imaging shows physical abnormalities in depressed brain. Medical Device Network 2019. https://www.medicaldevice-network.com/news/mri-for-depression/

26. Su L et al. Cerebral metabolism in major depressive disorder: a voxel-based meta-analysis of positron emission tomography studies. BMC Psychiatry 2014. https://bmcpsychiatry.biomedcentral.com/articles/10.1186/s12888-014-0321-9

27. Sheline YI et al. Resting-state functional MRI in depression unmasks increased connectivity between networks via the dorsal nexus. Proceedings of the

National Academy of Sciences of the United States of America 2010; 107: 11020–11025. https://www.ncbi.nlm.nih.gov/pmc/articles/PMC2890754/

28. Steiger A *et al.* Sleep encephalography as a biomarker in depression. Dove Press 2015; 5: 15–25. https://www.dovepress.com/sleep-electroencephalography-as-a-biomarker-in-depression-peer-reviewed-fulltext-article-CPT

29. Cleveland Clinic. Psychotherapy for depression. Cleveland Clinic 2018. https://my.clevelandclinic.org/health/treatments/9300--psychotherapy-for-depression

30. Zoppi L. What is music therapy and how does it work? Medical News Today 2020. https://www.medicalnewstoday.com/articles/music-therapy#for-depression

31. Cherry K. What is art therapy? VeryWell Mind 2021. https://www.verywellmind.com/what-is-art-therapy-2795755

32. Mayo Clinic Staff. Depression and anxiety: exercise eases symptoms. Mayo Clinic 2017. https://www.mayoclinic.org/diseases-conditions/depression/in-depth/depression-and-exercise/art-20046495

33. Johnson J. What foods are good for helping depression? Medical News Today 2019. https://www.medicalnewstoday.com/articles/318428

34. British National Health Service (NHS). Overview — Selective serotonin reuptake inhibitors (SSRIs). NHS 2021. https://www.nhs.uk/mental-health/talking-therapies-medicine-treatments/medicines-and-psychiatry/ssri-antidepressants/overview/

35. Leonard J. What to know about serotonin-norepinephrine reuptake inhibitor (SNRI) drugs. Medical News Today 2021. https://www.medicalnewstoday.com/articles/snri

36. Ankrom S. How MAOIs work and common side effects. VeryWell Mind 2020. https://www.verywellmind.com/monoamine-oxidase-inhibitors-maois-2584303

37. Ogbru A. Tricyclic antidepressants (TCAs). RxList 2021. https://www.rxlist.com/tricyclic_antidepressants_tcas/drug-class.htm

38. Pochwat B *et al.* An update on NMDA antagonists in depression. Expert Review of Neurotherapeutics 2019. https://pubmed.ncbi.nlm.nih.gov/31328587/

39. American Psychiatric Association. What is ElectroConvulsive Therapy (ECT)? American Psychiatric Association 2019. https://www.psychiatry.org/patients-families/ect

40. ScienceDaily. Long-term study data shows Deep Brain Stimulation (DBS) is effective treatment for most severe form of depression. ScienceDaily 2019. https://www.sciencedaily.com/releases/2019/10/191004074901.htm

41. Mayo Clinic Staff. Transcranial magnetic stimulation. Mayo Clinic 2018. https://www.mayoclinic.org/tests-procedures/transcranial-magnetic-stimulation/about/pac-20384625
42. Dryden-Edwards R. Suicide. MedicineNet, Inc 2021. https://www.medicinenet.com/suicide/article.htm
43. Caruso K. How to help. Suicide.org. http://www.suicide.org/how-to-talk-to-suicidal-callers.html
44. Centers for Disease Control and Prevention. COVID-19 coping with stress. Centers for Disease Control and Prevention 2022. https://www.cdc.gov/coronavirus/2019-ncov/daily-life-coping/managing-stress-anxiety.html
45. Duke-NUS Medical School. COVID-19: 1 in 3 adults anxious, depressed. Duke-NUS Medical School 2021. https://www.duke-nus.edu.sg/allnews/covid-19-1-in-3-adults-anxious-depressed
46. Wikipedia. Antidepressants and suicide risk. https://en.wikipedia.org/wiki/Antidepressants_and_suicide_risk
47. MentalHealthLiteracy.org. Teen Mental Health Speaks. Depression (download). MentalHealthLiteracy.org. https://mentalhealthliteracy.org/product/tmh-speaks-depression/

Appendix

Suicide help hotline (Singapore)

24-Hour Helpline: Samaritans of Singapore: 1 767
Samaritans of Singapore. https://www.sos.org.sg/
Samaritans of Singapore CareMail: pat@sos.org.sg

National Care Hotline: 1800-202-6868
(8am–12am daily, from 1 Sep 2020)

Mental well-being

— Fei Yue's Online Counselling Service
— Institute of Mental Health's Mental Health Helpline (6389-2222)
— Samaritans of Singapore (1800-221-4444)
— Silver Ribbon Singapore (6385-3714)

Marital and parenting issues

— Community Psychology Hub's Online Counselling platform

Violence or abuse

— Big Love Child Protection Specialist Centre (6445-0400)
— HEART @ Fei Yue Child Protection Specialist Centre (6819-9170)
— PAVE Integrated Services for Individual and Family Protection (6555-0390)
— Project StART (6476-1482)
— TRANS SAFE Centre (6449-9088)

Counselling

— TOUCHline (Counselling) – 1800 377 2252

18 Memory loss

Introduction[1]

The brain is the most complex structure in the known universe. It contains 86 billion neurons and 100 trillion connections between these neurons. For every second of our lives, thousands of nerve cells are firing off chemicals to control nearly every aspect of what we think or do. It is the damage of these nerve cells that can cause memory loss.

Causes of memory loss[2,3]

Memory loss is normal. None of us remember events that occur in the first few years of life. Even children over the age of four years have a rather erratic wandering memory. How then can we distinguish what is "normal" memory loss from "abnormal"? It is especially difficult to define abnormal memory loss in children.

Dementia is an umbrella term referring to memory loss in the elderly. Memory loss in children is not referred to as dementia; they do not get Alzheimer disease or other causes of dementia such as cardiovascular diseases. However, they do suffer memory loss caused by the following conditions:

1. Hypothyroidism[4]

The thyroid hormone accelerates all metabolic processes including brain development. Babies born with low thyroid levels will be slow intellectually and this can affect their memory.

2. **Parental neglect or abuse**[5]

The child's brain needs to be stimulated through love and care. If parents ignore the child who is seeking their attention, the kid will eventually not bother. If they do not receive positive stimulation from interactions with adults, they can feel lonely and remain silent. A worse situation occurs when a parent or caregiver abuses the child physically, psychologically or sexually. They may use physical violence like hitting or burning the child with boiling water or cigarettes, or shouting threatening words at the kid. All these actions will have severe effects on the child, making them have low self-esteem, feel depressed, anxious, fearful and develop behavioural disturbances such as aggression or violence. They will also suffer from memory loss.

3. **Depression**[6]

Some children experience depression for genetic reasons. Others become depressed because of environmental factors, such as child neglect, excessive physical punishment, or bullying at school. It is not uncommon for students to become depressed when they perform poorly in school exams or lose in sports competitions. Depressed children often have memory loss.

4. **Lack of sleep**[7]

Poor sleep or insomnia can result in poor memory. During both rapid eye movement as well as non-rapid eye movement sleep, memory is consolidated and strengthened. Children need about nine to 12 hours of sleep each day (see Chapter 8).

5. **Hunger**[8]

Hunger hinders one's ability to focus on studies and one's attention may be directed towards what food to eat. Erratic timing of meals can affect memory.

6. **Attention deficit hyperactivity disorder (ADHD)**[9]

People who suffer from ADHD cannot pay attention to their studies, and if their mind wanders, learning is impaired and there is short-term memory loss. They cannot remember their assignments, and they cannot finish homework and activities that need sustained attention. However, ADHD seems to have less effects on long-term memory.

7. **Dyslexia**[10]

Individuals with dyslexia have difficulty reading or writing. After reading a long passage, they feel that they have not read anything. They lose concentration and they cannot remember instructions or tasks.

8. **Poor diet and deficiency in vitamin B12 or folic acid**[11,12]

Some families have certain dietary exclusions which can result in vitamin and other deficiencies. Lack of vitamin B12 or folic acid is associated with memory loss.

9. **Trauma and head injuries**[13]

Following head trauma, one can suffer concussion and have memory loss. Fortunately most of the memory loss is transient, and it does not cause long-term problems. However, repeated head trauma, such as associated with certain sports like boxing, judo, karate, kickboxing, muay thai, rugby and soccer, can lead to memory loss. Excessive exposure to hot sun can cause heat stroke which damages the brain and impairs memory.

10. **Epilepsy and the side effects of antiepileptic medicine**[14]

Epilepsy has been described as an electrical storm in the brain. During an epileptic fit, any recent memory stored is wiped out. Several types of anti-epileptic medicine that "calm" brain activity can also reduce memory formation.

11. **Brain infections**[15]

Infections of the brain, such as meningitis or encephalitis, can lead to brain damage. This may lead to memory loss if not treated quickly.

12. **Brain tumours**[16]

Brain tumours, whether they are benign or malignant, or whether they originated from the brain or had spread from another part of the body, will lead to brain damage. This can cause loss of memory.

History taking[17]

While taking the history of a patient, one should concomitantly observe the behaviour of the child and their interactions with their parents or caregivers.

When did the parents first notice the memory loss? What things did the child forget? Was the memory loss of sudden or slow onset? Was it getting progressively worse or were there periods of normal memory? Did the child consistently forget to fulfil certain instructions? Was there any inappropriate behaviour? Has the memory loss affected schoolwork and family life? Is there any corroborative evidence from school teachers and other relatives? What sports does the child play? Was there any significant past illnesses, like severe infections or thyroid problems? What medicine is the child taking? Does the child fear school exams and suffer from depression?

One should sensitively try to explore whether or not there is any possibility of child abuse.

Examination

It is important to do a full general and neurological examination. The neurological examination includes how mentally alert the patient is, hearing and visual acuity, any tremors at rest, and jerky movements. There may be clues during the examination that the individual is emotionally depressed or highly anxious.

A cognitive assessment should be carried out as follows:

- Orientation — Do they know today's date, where are they now?
- Attention — Can they recite the months of the year or spell "BREAD" backwards?
- Memory — Can they give their home address or the name of the country's president?
- Language — Can they name items in a picture. Can they read a sentence from a passage and understand it?
- Executive function — The Stroop test asks what is the colour shown here: GREEN
- Praxis — Ask them to make alternating hand movements or imitate some gestures.
- Visuospatial function — Draw a clock face or overlapping pentagons.

These tests will help one decide if there is significant memory loss, and whether or not the patient needs to be referred to a psychologist for a more formal cognitive assessment.

Investigations[6]

Thyroid function, vitamin B12, folic acid, and cholesterol levels should be tested, and if human immunodeficiency virus (HIV-AIDS) or heavy metal poisoning is suspected, they should be tested as well.

A magnetic resonance imaging scan can show structural abnormalities and point towards Alzheimer disease, subdural haemorrhage, brain tumour, and other neurological conditions.

Management

The aims of management are several. Where possible, one treats the underlying disorder or diagnosis. For example, thyroxine is prescribed if hypothyroid is diagnosed. Similarly, vitamin B12 is administered if deficient. If there is epilepsy, head trauma, bleeding into the brain, or the presence of a brain tumour, these need to be treated appropriately.

To help a child with memory problems, here are some practical suggestions:

1. **Be patient**
   If your child forgets to follow instructions or leaves an important item at school, do not scold your child. Have patience, and encourage them to repeat the instructions several times. Have them write down the instructions to help as reminders.
2. **Shower love and attention**
   Give your child more attention and look at their positive attributes and achievements. Praise them when they succeed.
3. **Break instructions down into smaller steps**
   If your child has difficulty following multistep instructions, break them down into smaller more manageable steps. If the school homework or essay is too extensive, divide the assignment into smaller chunks and complete each part before moving onto the next.
4. **Create routines**
   Form patterns in regular daily activities and make it a regular routine. The same can be applied to learning how to tackle the writing of an essay or the solving of a maths problem.

How to improve memory in children[18-20]

Nonmedical activities that have been shown to delay or perhaps slightly improve memory loss. These include:

- Physical exercise: Walking, swimming, table tennis, tennis, yoga; avoid sports that might cause head trauma such as rugby, boxing, karate
- Social activities: Joining clubs; playing with other children; visiting parks, museums and art galleries; connecting with social media
- Mental exercise: Crossword puzzles, Sudoku, playing chess, learning a new language, photography, birdwatching, cooking, producing a TikTok video or a YouTube vlog, teaching others
- Music: Singing, playing an instrument, listening to favourite music, joining a choir or instrumental group, dancing, producing a video of the music performance
- Arts and crafts: Drawing, painting, woodwork, creating scrapbooks and photo albums
- Reading, writing, broadcasting: Starting a blog, writing a diary or a memoir, podcasting, writing on social media, making a vlog on travels and activities
- Computer games: Some stimulating computer games stimulate the brain. Try to limit the amount of time on the computer.

Conclusions[21]

Memory loss is one of the major problems of both the young and old. There are many causes, and if discovered and treated early, one might be able to mitigate some of the undesirable consequences. Currently, the best ways of slowing down memory loss is through nonmedical activities, including exercise, socialising, as well as arts and crafts.

References

1. Cherry K. How many neurons are in the brain? VeryWell Mind 2020. https://www.verywellmind.com/how-many-neurons-are-in-the-brain-2794889

2. Holmes J et al. Poor working memory: Impact and interventions. Advances in Child Development and Behavior 2010; 39: 1–43. https://www.sciencedirect.com/science/article/abs/pii/B9780123747488000019

3. THINK Neurology for Kids. What causes memory problems in children? THINK Neurology for Kids. https://www.thinkkids.com/blog/what-causes-memory-problems-in-children

4. Hereema E. Do thyroid disorders cause forgetfulness and brain fog? VeryWell Health 2022. https://www.verywellhealth.com/do-thyroid-disorders-cause-forgetfulness-98837

5. Romano LA. Childhood trauma and memory loss. Lisa A Romano 2018. https://www.lisaaromano.com/blog/childhood-trauma-and-memory-loss

6. Scaccia A. Can depression cause memory loss? Healthline 2019. https://www.healthline.com/health/depression/depression-and-memory-loss

7. Pacheco D. Memory and sleep. Sleep Foundation 2022. https://www.sleepfoundation.org/how-sleep-works/memory-and-sleep

8. Locwin B. Why is your memory so bad when you're hungry? Genetic Literacy Project 2016. https://geneticliteracyproject.org/2016/02/17/memory-bad-youre-hungry/

9. Watson K. ADHD and memory. Healthline 2021. https://www.healthline.com/health/adhd/adhd-memory

10. Swinton H. A quick guide to dyslexia and working memory issues. Defeat Dyslexia 2016. http://www.defeat-dyslexia.com/2016/04/a-quick-guide-to-dyslexia-and-working-memory/

11. Cross M. Vitamin B12 memory loss and dementia. Medium 2020. https://medium.com/feed-your-brain/vitamin-b12-memory-loss-and-dementia-e0879d34ce02

12. Pathways Home Health and Hospice. Folic acid and memory loss. Pathways Home Health and Hospice. https://pathwayshealth.org/hospice-topics/folic-acid-and-memory-loss-what-you-should-know/

13. Hart T & Sander A. Memory and traumatic brain injury. Model Systems Knowledge Translation Center 2016. https://msktc.org/tbi/factsheets/Memory-And-Traumatic-Brain-Injury

14. Eddy CM et al. The cognitive impact of antiepileptic drugs. Therapeutic Advances in Neurological Disorders 2011; 4: 385–407. https://www.ncbi.nlm.nih.gov/pmc/articles/PMC3229254/

15. Wilson B. Managing memory problems after encephalitis. Encephalitis Society 2020. https://www.encephalitis.info/managing-memory-problems-after-encephalitis

16. Wolf MC. Brain tumors and memory loss.Memory-Loss-Facts.com. https://www.memory-loss-facts.com/brain-tumors.html

17. D'Alessandro DM. What can cause memory problems? Pediatric Education 2011. https://pediatriceducation.org/2011/11/07/what-can-cause-memory-problems/

18. Jacobson R. How to help kids with working memory issues. Child Mind Institute. https://childmind.org/article/how-to-help-kids-with-working-memory-issues/

19. Tian C. Short term memory loss in children: causes and tips to cope with it. First Cry Parenting 2018. https://parenting.firstcry.com/articles/short-term-memory-loss-in-children-causes-and-tips-to-cope-with-it/

20. Dewar G. Working memory in children. Parenting Science 2019. https://parentingscience.com/working-memory/

21. Farrer TH, Eifert EK. Dementia and Memory. Wiley 2022. ISBN 1119658098

19 Dyscalculia

Introduction

A small number of children do badly in mathematics in school. For a child above the age of seven, most are expected to be able to count backwards mentally, doubling or halving numbers, doing simple multiplication, and performing complex procedures like long division. Taking too long, or failing to perform these actions can be due to a condition known as dyscalculia.

Definition[1,2]

Dyscalculia is a learning disability with impairment in understanding arithmetic, such as difficulty in knowing how to manipulate numbers and perform mathematical calculations, as well as learning mathematical facts. The level of performance is lower than expected for age and educational experiences.

Symptoms of dyscalculia[3]

- Difficulty counting forwards and backwards
- Not knowing which number is smaller or larger
- Difficulty memorising the multiplication table
- Confusing maths symbols and signs
- Difficulty telling the time
- Being late for appointments, not able to keep track of time
- Often reads or writes numbers incorrectly

- Difficulty understanding and remembering math concepts
- Difficulty with spatial orientation which can manifest as incorrect map-reading or following directions.

Epidemiology[4]

The prevalence of dyscalculia is estimated to be between 3 and 7 per cent of the population.

Diagnosis[5]

To date, there has not been a consensus on the appropriate diagnostic criteria for dyscalculia. Therefore, several diagnostic tests are employed using different measurements. A direct face-to-face assessment interview is essential in arriving at a diagnosis.

The diagnosis is often missed because children who do poorly in mathematics are accepted as being on the lower part of the bell curve. Parents and teachers sometimes assume that these children are less intelligent, and therefore do poorly with handling numbers.

Causes[6]

Identical twin studies showed that the concordance rate of dyscalculia is 58 per cent, whereas in dizygotic twins, it is 39 per cent. Dyscalculia runs in families, and therefore, there must be a genetic cause. It is also found in some people with Turner Syndrome, where there is a missing X-chromosome. However, in cases of dyscalculia without a family history, we presume that the environment plays a part in the cause, but this has not been identified yet.

Aptitude vs ability

""Aptitude" is defined as an inborn potential to perform certain tasks, and "ability" is the learnt or acquired skills. In other words, "aptitude" is an innate natural flair that one is born with; in contrast, "ability" is developed through constant practice. Individuals with dyscalculia are born with the inability to handle numbers, hence theirs is a negative "aptitude". However, they are able to do well in other subjects like literature, geography, and history.

Comorbidities[7]

There are many reasons why some children struggle with mathematics. These include the co-existence with dyslexia where a child may have difficulty understanding the words or symbols used in a maths problem. Others may have attention deficit hyperactivity disorder (ADHD) and cannot pay attention, so the mind wanders halfway through a maths problem. Or they may have auditory processing difficulties. If a child comes from a disadvantaged family that does not introduce arithmetic to the young child, then that individual may have problems with simple arithmetic.

Children who do not have dyscalculia, but have the other learning problems like dyslexia, ADHD, or come from a disadvantaged social or educational background, can still retain their aptitude for mathematics. Hence, these children will maintain their ability in picking up mathematics at a normal rate, which is faster compared to individuals with dyscalculia. The latter will find it harder to improve their mathematics capabilities. This is one of the techniques used by psychologists and educationalists to help diagnose dyscalculia, and distinguish it from other conditions (dyslexia, ADHD, poor social environment) that may be mistaken and misdiagnosed as dyscalculia.

Tips for parents on how to manage dyscalculia[8]

The following are tips that you can try to help your child better learn and understand maths and hopefully raise their self-esteem.

- Allow them to use their fingers, a calculator or a mobile device when they count, add or subtract
- Allow them to use a tablet computer or paper with ruled lines or graph paper to help keep columns and numbers straight and neat
- Use music or dance to a beat to teach maths

- Use visual aids and draw pictures to help solve maths word problems
- Praise them for effort and hard work, and not the outcome
- Discuss with them about their learning disability
- Teach them ways to cope with anxiety
- Discover your child's other abilities like love of words or practical abilities and help develop them

Practical classroom management

Talk to the teachers privately about your child's dyscalculia and their educational needs. You may want to request for the following:

- A quiet workspace
- Allow them to use a mobile device or calculator during maths class and tests
- Give extra time for tests
- If potentially helpful, record the lectures

Conclusions

Dyscalculia is a common condition affecting 3 to 7 per cent of the population and is often missed because performing poorly in mathematics is accepted in many schools and families. Early diagnosis can help give the individual educational and psychological support. Further research into the causes and potential methods of improving this condition is being undertaken. We hope that we can find ways to help these individuals.

References

1. Wikipedia. Dyscalculia. https://en.wikipedia.org/wiki/Dyscalculia
2. Cognifit Research. Dyscalculia in Children. Cognifit Research 2019. https://www.cognifit.com/pathology/dyscalculia
3. Jacobson R. How to spot dyscalculia. Child Mind Institute. https://childmind.org/article/how-to-spot-dyscalculia/
4. Haberstroh S & Schulte-Körne G. The Diagnosis and Treatment of Dyscalculia Deutsches Arzteblatt International 2019; 116: 107–14. https://www.ncbi.nlm.nih.gov/pmc/articles/PMC6440373/

5. Miller K. What Is Dyscalculia? WebMD 2021. https://www.webmd.com/add-adhd/childhood-adhd/dyscalculia-facts

6. Singh M. Role of genetics in prevalence of dyscalculia. https://numberdyslexia.com/role-of-genetics-in-prevalence-of-dyscalculia/

7. Living with dyslexia: What are some co-occurring conditions? http://livingwithdyslexia.in/what-are-some-co-occuring-conditionslearning-difficulties/

8. WOW Parenting. What is dyslexia? 7 Ways to help your child deal with it. https://wowparenting.com/blog/ways-to-deal-with-dyscalculia/

20 Screen time

Introduction[1]

About half the children who are going to develop mental illnesses will start before the age of 14. One of the major contributors to disorders of mental health is spending too much time with television, computers, handphones, and constantly playing video games.

We realise that digital technology is a double-edged sword. On the one hand it helps enhance communication and learning and is a great source of entertainment and relaxation. On the other hand it has adverse effects. Spending too much screen time robs one of the opportunities to interact with family and friends, or undertake physical activities, or engage in music or the arts. It can be psychologically traumatic, addictive and deprive one of beauty sleep. Watching inappropriately violent or pornographic videos can lead to unacceptable behaviours. Some Internet messages and videos contain toxic materials that result in cyberbullying.

Symptoms of negative mental effects of the internet[2,3]

Adverse mental effects of the Internet differ from one person to another. They range from mild symptoms to severe behavioural problems. Here are some of the warning signs:

- Feeling lonely
- Anxiety

- Poor sleep
- Low self-esteem
- Impulsivity
- Attention deficit, poor concentration
- Deteriorating schoolwork
- Reduced appetite and weight loss
- Extreme mood swings
- Personality changes
- Feeling sad, withdrawn, depressed
- Attempting self-harm or hurting others
- Risky behaviour

Parenting controls

Parents or caregivers have to take the initiative and control screentime and content of the programmes. It is recommended that children under the age of two should not be allowed to use laptops or handphones. From two to four years of age, it is recommended that screentime should not exceed one hour a day. Above the age of four, children may be allowed to watch videos up to two hours a day.

Harmful content, excessive violence, and pornography should be filtered out. There are programmes nowadays that can determine which are whitelist and which are blacklist programmes and filter the latter. But even with these auto-filters, parents and caregivers should keep track of the child's online activities and stop them watching undesirable materials.

Gaming addiction[4,5]

With closure of schools during COVID-19 lockdowns, children may have little to do at home, and this has resulted in an increase in the number of children indulging in online gaming, and an increase in the number of hours spent playing these games.

This has detrimental effects over time. For example, so much time is spent with these games that less time is devoted to social interaction with parents and friends. Less time is spent on physical exercise, art, music, dance, and other hobbies. Penned up at home, some children become irritable, moody, and depressed.

Many studies have shown that during the COVID-19 pandemic, the time children spend playing computer games increased by more than 30 per cent, and the gaming industry worldwide has also seen an upsurge in sales. Some become addicted.

There is uncertainty whether playing computer games can help or adversely affect children. Some reports claim that video games are exciting and keep the child occupied without which they will be bored. Others suggest that perhaps spending too much time playing these games can cause the following:

- Decline in school performance
- Cause deterioration in relationships
- Social isolation
- Staying up very late and causing sleep deprivation
- Poor nutrition resulting in poor health
- Obesity due to overeating junk food

Cyberbullying[6]

During the early months of COVID-19 pandemic, there was an increase in cyberbullying. Three studies have shown a slight decrease as the pandemic dragged on. Unfortunately, this online bullying does not seem to be eradicated, hence, it is important to be aware of these activities and to counsel the child or refer them to a counsellor.

Alternative activities

For younger children, parents may have more control and take their kids out for walks, do sports and art, play games and music, dance or read books. Simply engaging in conversation with your child or going shopping together will reduce time on computers and handphones.

Final note

If your child displays any mental health problems, do not delay in consulting a counsellor, a paediatrician, or a clinical psychologist who specialises in handling these problems.

We are not saying that you should deny your child the use of computers, handphones or mobile games. It is almost impossible to do that in this day and age. We want to create an environment where one can spend some time using digital technology, but we also want to balance that with other activities like interacting with family and friends, doing physical activities and engaging in the arts. The objective is to promote positive mental health in your child who will then grow up to be an outstanding adult.

References

1. Newsweek Amplify. Is the internet harming the mental health of children? Newsweek 2020. https://www.newsweek.com/amplify/internet-harming-mental-health-children
2. Organization for Economic Cooperation and Development. Children and young people's mental health in the digital age. Organization for Economic Cooperation and Development 2018. https://www.oecd.org/els/health-systems/Children-and-Young-People-Mental-Health-in-the-Digital-Age.pdf
3. Children's Bureau. Effects of technology on mental health. Children's Bureau 2019 https://www.all4kids.org/news/blog/effects-of-technology-on-mental-health/
4. Analytics Insight. Gaming boom in COVID-19 times. Analytics Insight 2020. https://www.analyticsinsight.net/gaming-boom-in-covid-19-times-analysis-insights/
5. Peterson TJ. How many hours of video games is too much? HealthyPlace Inc 2020. https://www.healthyplace.com/addictions/gaming-disorder/how-many-hours-of-video-games-is-too-much
6. Patchin JW. Bullying during the COVID-19 pandemic. Cyberbullying Research Center 2021. https://cyberbullying.org/bullying-during-the-covid-19-pandemic

21 COVID-19 pandemic effects on mental health

Introduction

COVID-19 has swept through the entire world causing deaths as well as serious medical and psychological problems upsetting the economy of many countries. Furthermore, the virus keeps on mutating, making it almost impossible to get rid of.

The earlier variants of COVID-19 did not affect children as much as older people. The newer mutations, like the Omicron variant, is affecting larger numbers of unvaccinated children. Direct infection by the virus causes less severe symptoms compared to the Delta variant. However, the Omicron variant is far more transmissible, and because a larger number of people are infected, it is causing major problems in the healthcare services for both children and adults.

The neuropsychological effects of COVID-19 on children can be due to the direct effect of the virus on the brain, or secondary to the body's immune response to the virus, or it can be the result of measures taken by the authorities to curb the spread of the virus.

Why and how has the pandemic affected the mental health of children?

Physical signs and symptoms of COVID-19 infection[1]

The coronavirus responsible is airborne and spreads from one person to another by droplets when breathing out or coughing. There is a wide spectrum of symptoms ranging from barely any at all, to the full house affecting nearly every organ in the body. Common manifestations are fever, coughing, breathlessness, sore throat, runny nose and a loss of smell and taste. Appetite may be diminished and there may be abdominal discomfort, drowsiness, and weakness. Some children have severe respiratory symptoms leading to them turning blue and requiring oxygen and assisted ventilation. Others may have inflammation of the heart or myocarditis. Adults' minds may manifest a confused haze and they may become delirious and begin hallucinating. These mental symptoms uncommonly develop in children. Luckily, the life-threatening signs of COVID-19 are also much rarer in fully vaccinated children.

Lockdowns and other restrictions[2]

In an attempt to curb the spread and to cope with the ravages of COVID-19, governments have imposed a number of rules and regulations. This varies widely from minimal guidelines to very strict directives. Enforcement of the decrees also differs quite widely from country to country. In general, Asian countries tend to be stricter and more diligent in enforcing the regulations, and punish transgressions with harsher penalties. The measures initially introduced were relatively mild and these included the wearing of face masks, social distancing, and the frequent washing of hands.

But these measures did not stop the virus spreading. More severe directives were instigated by governments, including imposing lockdowns. This meant that people had to stay at home and were only allowed out for essential activities, like buying food or seeing a doctor. Schools and most offices, shops selling non-essential goods, airports, hotels, theatres and cinemas, gyms, restaurants and other businesses were closed.

These measures led to a severe slowing down of the economy, and many businesses closing shop. Unemployment shot up, and many families struggled to cope with the drop in income. Certain industries have been harder hit than others, and this included tourism, hospitality, arts, entertainment and leisure businesses.

Effects on children[3-5]

There was a rise in the number of consultations for counselling and psychological support. The incidence of depression and suicide increased after the start of the pandemic especially in adolescents.

Most children have been affected quite badly when day care centres, kindergartens and schools were closed or the hours of attendance drastically reduced. This resulted in less opportunities for them to physically interact with their classmates and teachers. Many children actually looked forward to going to school and they brightened up when interacting with their peers. They learnt better in a classroom setting and were better motivated to learn because of competition with their classmates.

Cooped up at home for long periods of time had different effects on different children. There were some beneficial effects resulting from increased contact of a child with their parents, which led to greater communication with their loved ones. Sensitive, caring caretakers knew how to help their children improve their mental health. On the other hand, the opposite also occurred: some parents were less tolerant and admonished their children at the slightest transgression of family rules. For example, if such a parent saw their child playing games, using their handphone, or watching TV, they disciplined them and the conflict it created led to temper tantrums, anxiety and even depression.

Online learning at home flourished during the pandemic, and physical exercises dropped. Official studies showed that obesity rose by more than 10 per cent in Singapore, and poverty and food insecurity escalated in poorer countries.

Non-academic activities including sports, art, music, dance, and theatre were also curtailed in a number of schools. This led to two serious mental problems: anxiety and depression. Identification of these two emotional problems early on enabled timely intervention to be instituted. The early signs of these disturbances are listed below:

Early signs of anxiety include:

- Feeling very nervous or tense
- Feeling restless or feeling on edge
- Feeling excessively tired
- Sleep disturbances
- Asking for repeated reassurance "are you sure it is safe to do this"
- Irritable, aggressive, temper tantrums, meltdowns
- Social withdrawal
- Less physically active, more sedentary
- Playing outside less

- Excessive online screentime
- Tightness of muscle or muscle cramps
- Palpitations of the heart
- Abdominal discomfort
- Sweating more profusely

Early signs of depression include:

- Reduced appetite
- Sleep problems
- Poor mental concentration and not paying attention
- Reduced self-esteem and self-confidence
- Ideas of guilt and unworthiness
- Social withdrawal
- Harbouring thoughts of self-harm or suicide

If identified early, one can intervene, and if necessary, refer these children for counselling.

Autism spectrum children[6,7]

Children on the autism spectrum were affected by COVID-19 because when schools were closed and they were isolated at home, their normal routines were disrupted. Unable to attend school physically or have direct contact with peers, teachers and therapists, they were stuck at home, and many felt lonely and became more stressed and anxious. It should be noted that there was the occasional child who was not so badly affected by changes in routine, and even enjoyed their home environment.

Caregivers can do the following to help autistic children cope better at home:

- Try to explain why there are changes in their routine, using visual explanations where possible
- Draw out a new routine, allow the child to make choices
- Be consistent
- Allow rest periods between each activity
- Draw out times for meals, snacks and drinks

- Use different coping strategies, such as listening to music, counting 1 to 10, drawing pictures, going for a walk, exercising, taking deep breaths
- Visit less crowded places like gardens, zoos, museums, and shopping centres
- Make time for social connections whenever possible
- Regulate access to screen time

Children with Attention Deficit Hyperactivity Disorder (ADHD)[8,9]

Children with ADHD are more likely than their peers to be vulnerable to the emotional afflictions of COVID-19. Many families lacked preparedness for school closures or restrictions during the pandemic.

ADHD individuals often complained of difficulties with remote learning. The reduction in face-to-face interactions led to feelings of isolation, loneliness, boredom and depression. Their motivation to accomplish tasks was decreased. The standard of their schoolwork dropped significantly. They displayed sleep problems, anxieties, irritability, family conflicts, rule-breaking behaviour, temper tantrums and physical aggression. When going out to playgrounds, shops, and museums, ADHD children sometimes had difficulty maintaining social distancing or wearing masks, so they were more exposed and the virus could spread more readily.

Some children with ADHD had increased behavioural problems during the COVID-19 pandemic. It is advisable to consult a doctor for advice on management.

Vaccine hesitancy is encountered when it comes to deciding whether or not children with ADHD should receive the COVID-19 vaccine. The consensus of medical opinion is that vaccines should be given.

Prevention and treatment of mental health issues

Below are listed some of the actions that caregivers can take to promote mental health and prevent problems such as anxiety, depression, and gaming addiction:

- Socialise more and talk more to friends and loved ones
- Encourage regular physical exercise or sports, go out for a walk
- Develop other hobbies e.g. art, music, dance, theatre performance, writing
- Read books
- Play board games and puzzles
- Reduce screen time to less than one hour per day for kindergarten children, less than two hours per day for school-aged children
- Structure time for schoolwork and play
- Take a break between game levels
- Healthy diet: avoid junk food, do not overeat
- Keep a pet
- Yoga, meditation, mindfulness practice
- Regular health check-ups
- Watch for warning signs of anxiety, depression, gaming addiction, and ask for help before it is too late
- Empower your child to overcome negative thoughts and feelings: "You are stronger than you feel"
- Validate your child's concerns and feelings. Tell them: "It is OK to be upset"
- Avoid focusing on the worry
- Limit exposure to the media or the news because bad news can be depressing
- Be mindful of the conversations you have with other family members because the child can overhear what is said
- Create daily routines that gives your child predictability and control
- Create a comfortable environment for your child
- Avoid substance abuse
- Do not discriminate against people with mental disorders

Racial tensions

Reports of racist incidents increased during the COVID-19 pandemic. East Asians bore the brunt of the abuse. They were accused of bringing the "China virus" to their country. There were verbal invectives and physical violence in the streets, shopping centres, and schools. Children were especially terrified by these unexpected attacks. Gradually, the number of xenophobic incidents and hate crimes has diminished.

Conclusions[10]

COVID-19 has changed everyone's lives, and it does not appear to be going away any time soon. Children are affected both physically and mentally. Be sensitive to any changes in their mood or activities. Underlying conditions like autism and ADHD can cause one to respond differently to the pandemic. There has been an increase in gaming addiction since the start of COVID-19, and this can cause further psychological problems including depression. Discuss the emotional problems with the children, and consult or refer them to a counsellor early, before the condition turns into a tragedy.

References

1. Mayo Clinic Staff. COVID-19 in babies and children. Mayo Clinic 2022. https://www.mayoclinic.org/diseases-conditions/coronavirus/in-depth/coronavirus-in-babies-and-children/art-20484405

2. Dalabih A et al. The COVID-19 pandemic and pediatric mental health. Nature Pediatric Research 2022. https://www.nature.com/articles/s41390-022-01952-w

3. Tomi B et al. Sounding the alarm for children's mental health during the COVID-19 pandemic. JAMA Pediatrics 2022. https://jamanetwork.com/journals/jamapediatrics/fullarticle/2788911

4. Ford T et al. The Impact of COVID-19 on the mental health of children and young people. The Conversation Dec 2021. https://theconversation.com/the-impact-of-covid-19-on-the-mental-health-of-children-and-young-people-in-the-uk-what-the-research-says-172653

5. Abramson A. Children's mental health is in crisis. American Psychological Association 2022; 53: 69. https://www.apa.org/monitor/2022/01/special-childrens-mental-health

6. Lugo-Marin J et al. COVID-19 effects in people with autism spectrum disorder and their caregivers. Research in Autism Spectrum Disorders 2021; 83: 101757. https://www.ncbi.nlm.nih.gov/pmc/articles/PMC7904459/

7. Salomon SH. 5 Things People With Autism and Their Caregivers Should Know About COVID-19 Vaccines. Everyday Health 2021. https://www.everydayhealth.com/autism/things-people-with-autism-and-caregivers-should-know-about-covid-19-vaccines/

8. Rosenthal E *et al.* Impact of COVID-19 on youth with ADHD. Sage Journals 2021. https://journals.sagepub.com/doi/10.1177/10870547211063641

9. Nigg J. Mental health, ADHD, and COVID-19. Psychology Today 2021. https://www.psychologytoday.com/us/blog/helping-kids-through-adhd/202104/mental-health-adhd-and-covid-19

10. Toms S. COVID-19: Singapore schools tackle mental health amid pandemic stress. BBC News 2021. https://www.bbc.com/news/world-asia-56720368

Index